B

Conceptual Modelling in Computational Immunology

Martina Husáková

ʙ

2015

Published in the Czech Republic by Tomáš Bruckner, Řepín – Živonín, 2015
Academic Series

This book was reviewed by
doc. Ing. Petr Hájek, Ph.D., University of Pardubice
Ing. Pavel Čech, Ph.D., University of Hradec Králové
Dr. Ing. Ján Vaščák, Technical University of Košice

Visit us at http://pub.bruckner.cz

ISBN 978-80-87924-00-6 (hardcover)
ISBN 978-80-87924-01-3 (paperback, print on demand)
ISBN 978-80-87924-02-0 (pdf e-book)

DEDICATION

I dedicate this monograph to Ladislav, Radka and Denny for their loving support, patience and empathy.

ACKNOWLEDGEMENTS

This monograph was supported by the project No. CZ.1.07/2.3.00/30.0052 - Development of Research at the University of Hradec Králové with the participation of postdocs, financed from EU (ESF project).

I would like to thank to Vanda Pickett for proofreading all parts of the manuscript and her valuable comments and helpful advices in writing this monograph.

INVESTICE DO ROZVOJE VZDĚLÁVÁNÍ

Abstract

Computational immunology is a subarea of computational biology aiming at the investigation of the complexity of the natural immune system with the assistance of computer science, mathematics, physics, and data analysis. Complexity of the natural immune system complicates exploration of immune processes and their understanding with traditional in vivo or in vitro strategies. Computational immunology brings in silico approaches where models and simulations can offer deeper insight into the hardly investigated natural immune system. Modelling of complex systems requires analysis of the problem and application domain that is going to be covered by the models. Conceptual modelling helps with representation of the most important "players" most likely responsible for the investigated behaviour together with the relationships between them. These conceptual models are used for programming of the computational models that are used for simulations. The help of experts is necessary during conceptualisation and simulations. The expert helps with the identification of the crucial biological entities and interactions between them, and guides the "modeller" towards the correct conceptual model. Results of simulations should be evaluated by the expert to determine whether the simulations offer added value for the understanding of the investigated problem.

This monograph is focused on computational immunology in the view of conceptualisation of particular immune processes. The most cited approaches of conceptual modelling in computational immunology are mentioned and compared. This monograph is mainly concerned with the conceptualisation of selected immune processes occurring in the lymph node, with the use of the AML (Agent Modelling Language). The AML is an extension of the standardised UML language in terms of the multi-agent systems. The natural immune system is viewed as the multi-agent system consisting of autonomous entities – artificial agents – immune cells.

CONTENTS

1. INTRODUCTION

Progress of computational technologies represents a significant contribution to the study of complex systems. J. L. Singer, the specialist in the field of complex systems, describes a complex system as a whole composed of many interacting agents with non-linear behaviour. This behaviour cannot be deduced from the behaviour of individual agents in the system (Morowitz and Singer, 1995). Complexity science investigates components of complex systems, relations and interactions between them together with rules managing their behaviour. Typical examples of complex systems are: ecosystems, climate, social network, telecommunication infrastructure, global network like Internet, metabolic networks or neural networks. These systems are studied in depth within various research areas and projects. This monograph focuses on the investigation of the amazing complexity of the natural immune system through various conceptual approaches. Special attention is paid to the approach used in conjunction with the multi-agent systems – The Agent Modelling Language (AML). The natural immune system is a complex and adaptive system ensuring the homeostasis in the inner environment of the living system. Complexity of this system is mainly caused by the amount of "players" and relations between them. The non-linear and dynamic nature of the natural immune system (NIS) renders its behaviour far from predictable. This fact complicates the investigation of the immunity. The immunity appears in various research disciplines, see Fig. 1:

- Immunological computation (Artificial immune systems) uses immunity only as an inspiration for solving various problems arising from different application domains (e. g. in computer security, scheduling, optimization, decision making or pattern recognition) (Cohen, 2007), (Timmis et al., 2008).
- Immuno-computing is focused on hardware implementation of principles appearing in the natural immune system (Cohen, 2007), (Timmis et al., 2008). The aim is to develop "immune-computer" that should behave similarly as the natural immune system (Tarakanov et al., 2005). This initiative is often combined with the immunological computation (de Castro, 2006).
- Computational immunology (Immuno-informatics) uses techniques of computational science, modelling, simulation, mathematics, data analysis, physics, for better understanding of processes occurring inside the NIS (Garrett, 2005), (Timmis et al., 2008).
- Immunological bioinformatics applies methods of bioinformatics in immunology (Lund et al., 2005).

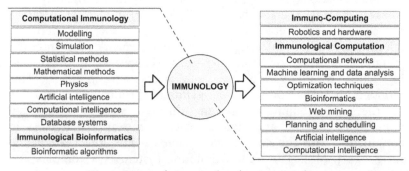

Fig. 1: Research areas related to immunology

At present, artificial immune systems and computational immunology are the main strands in the field of study where immunity and computational science meet. This monograph focuses on the subarea of computational biology (CB) - computational immunology (CI). It concentrates mainly on conceptual modelling of various immune properties and processes.

It is obvious that the natural immune system is very complex. Conceptual models can help with this complexity, but some abstraction is inevitable. Conceptual models are an important part of the development of immune simulators. Immune simulators can became useful tools for discovering new principles or rules governing the natural immune system. The primary goal is to investigate the Agent Modelling Language for conceptualisation of the immune processes occurring in the lymph node – one of the best known immune organs. These conceptual models are going to be used for a development of the immune system simulator of the lymph node, i. e. for visualisation of interactions occurring in various parts of this organ.

If we want to investigate the natural immune system with the help of computational science techniques or try to develop immunity-inspired algorithms, it is necessary to understand how the natural immune system behaves. The second chapter introduces the fundamental principles of the innate and the adaptive immunity. These principles are important for understanding the following chapters. The third chapter focuses on the study and application of immune principles for development of immunity-based algorithms, because the term artificial immune system has a historical relation to the computational immunology. The fourth chapter introduces computational immunology from a historical point of view. Approaches to immunity modelling and future perspectives of this research area are also presented. The fifth chapter focuses on the CoSMoS process as a framework for development of complex system models and simulations. The sixth chapter presents conceptual techniques which can be used for specification of conceptual models of the natural immune system. This chapter also mentions a comparison of these conceptual techniques. The Agent Modelling Language is introduced in the seventh chapter. Examination of the use of the Agent Modelling Language for computational immunology is mentioned in the eight chapter where it is applied for conceptualisation of particular immune processes occurring in the lymph node. Contributiveness of the AML is presented in the ninth chapter. Final remarks are presented in the tenth chapter, together with the conclusion.

2. Natural Immune System

The natural immune system (NIS) is a complex and adaptive system ensuring the homeostasis in the inner environment of the living system. Complexity of the system is mainly caused by the amount of "players" and relations between them. The non-linear and dynamic nature of the system renders the behaviour far from predictable. The NIS is an ambient system, because it does not have the centre for coordination or cooperation of its activities. The NIS is highly interconnected system with other complex systems, especially the endocrine, nervous and reproductive system. Redundancy is one of the fundamental principles of the NIS. The NIS does not tend to fail due to the small disturbances. Distinguishing between dangerous and safe objects is one of the main tasks of the natural immune system. These objects are often referred to as antigens. They can be defined as objects with the ability to initiate the activity of the NIS. They can come from the outer environment – non-self antigens (viruses, bacteria, fungi, parasites, etc.) or from the inner environment – self-antigens (an old or a damaged cell). Self and safe antigens are not under an attack from the NIS in the case of a correct behaviour of the NIS. Sometimes the NIS is not in a correct state. Autoimmune diseases are a result of a wrong behaviour of the NIS when the NIS damages biological components which are parts of the body. Stabilization mechanisms are crucial for the maintenance of homeostasis and the survival of the organism. The characteristics important for ensuring the stability of the organism are (de Castro and Timmis, 2002), (Timmis, 2007):

- Memory: If the NIS meets antigens several times it is able to react against them faster and more thoroughly in comparison with the first encounter.
- Adaptation: Immune cells go through various structural changes resulting in their ability to play various roles in the NIS.
- Diversity: The NIS is able to react with diverse antigens.
- Decentralization: The NIS does not have the centre which could be responsible for regulating all immune processes.
- Robustness and fault tolerance: An organism can exist even if some faults occur within it, but the NIS tries to eliminate these potential danger events as much as possible.
- Self-organisation: Immune cells can be in the right place at the right time. The cytokines (communication molecules) play important role in this process. They influence self-organisation principles of immune cells for homeostasis maintenance.

2.1   Natural immune system as a layered system

The natural immune system can be perceived as a layered system. First of all, exo-antigens meet the non-immunological layer. This layer contains mechanical, chemical and microbial barriers trying to eliminate a danger in the first line of defence. If these barriers are not effective the exo-antigen encounters the innate layer of the natural immune system. Innate immune system is the second line of defence after the danger has entered the body through the skin. This layer is composed of immune cells which are able to react against antigens very quickly (in minutes) (Abbas and Lichtman, 2010). Immune cells of the innate immune system are not able to remember antigens from the past. Adaptive layer of the natural immune system is the third line of defence. It is more specific and slower in comparison to the innate immunity (Abbas and Lichtman, 2010). It reacts against antigens in hours, days or weeks. Specificity of the adaptive NIS is based on the ability of the immune cells to remember antigens and to react faster in case of repeated conflicts with these antigens. Fig. 2 depicts the NIS as a layered system consisting of the innate and adaptive layer.

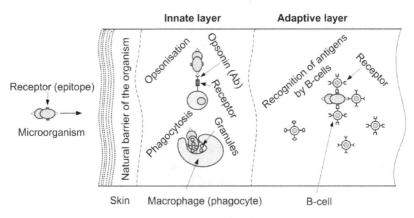

Fig. 2: Innate and adaptive immune system

2.2 Immune cells of the natural immune system

The natural immune system uses heterogeneous "army of soldiers" – immune cells which originate in the bone marrow as hematopoietic stem cells. Two main classes of immune cells are then formed: myeloid and lymphoid stem cells, see Fig. 3 (adopted and adjusted from (Todar [n. d.])). Myeloid lineage of immune cells plays key role in the innate immunity, see the subchapter 2.1. Polymorphonuclear leukocytes (e. g. basophils, neutrophils or monocytes) are typical examples of the innate layer of the NIS (Murphy et al., 2008). Dendritic cells, macrophages and monocytes are antigen presenting cells (APC). They can present antigenic peptides to other immune cells, especially T-cells (lymphoid immune cells). Lymphoid lineage of immune cells ensures the adaptive immunity. White-blood cells (lymphocytes) are representatives of this lineage and are one of the most important types of immune cells of the NIS. B-cells develop and mature in the bone marrow. Maturation continues in the secondary lymphatic organs after encountering with antigens. Plasmatic form is the final stage of the B-cells. Plasmatic B-cells produce antibodies which are aimed at antigens. Memory form is the second possible stage of the B-cells. Memory B-cells are able to remember antigens and can be more effective in the future against these antigens. T-cells develop in the bone marrow, like B-cells, but they mature in the thymus.

They can recognise antigenic peptides only with the assistance of the APC which present these peptides on their surface. B-cells can recognise antigens directly – without this assistance. T-cells can have different final stages (Murphy et al., 2008), (Abbas et al., 2011):

- T_c-cells ($T_{cytotoxic}$-cells): They eliminate dangerous "objects" in the organism. They have suppressive function in the NIS.
- T_h-cells (T_{helper}-cells): They help with the recognition of antigens and the induction of an immune response. They have regulatory function in the NIS.
- T_{sup}-cells/T_{req}-cells ($T_{suppressor}$-cells, $T_{regulatory}$-cells): They inhibit immune response of B-cells, T_h-cells or T_c-cells.

Cells of the Immune System

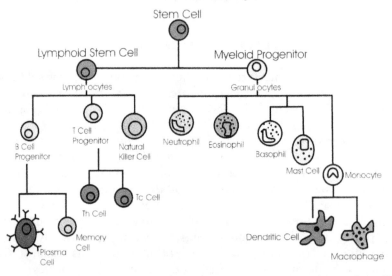

Fig. 3: Cells of the immune system (adopted and adjusted from (Todar [n. d.]))

2.3 MOLECULES OF THE NATURAL IMMUNE SYSTEM

One of the main functions of the immune cells is the ability to recognise "objects" which can be potentially dangerous for the organism. This recognition is realised through various surface structures (molecules) of immune cells. Immune cells have various surface structures which are used for their classification, see illustration on Fig. 4 where various surface structures of T-cells and B-cells with their ligands (CD28 – CD80, CD40L – CD40, FAS-L – FAS, TCR – MHC-II and BCR) are depicted. Some of them play the role of adhesive molecules which are able to ensure connections between cells or to bind the cell to the antigen for transferring information about the antigen into the cell. Surface molecules change their character during development of the immune cell. Some of them are present in the initial phases of life of these immune cells, others occur later during development. Antigenic receptors are able to detect antigens with direct binding (B-cells) or with the help of antigen-presenting cells (APC) containing MHC (Major histocompatibility complex, HLA (Human leukocyte antigen) in case of human) surface molecules which bind to the antigen (Sompayrac, 2012). Antigenic receptor of the T-cell is then bound to the MHC surface molecule of the APC. Recognition of surface structures can be demonstrated with the key-lock metaphor.

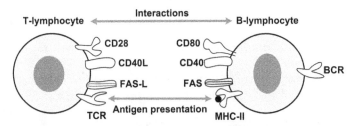

Fig. 4: Surface structures of immune cells - example of T-cell and B-cell

2.4 IMMUNE ORGANS OF THE NATURAL IMMUNE SYSTEM

Immune cells develop and mature in the primary immune organs of the natural immune system. Bone marrow and thymus play the role of primary immune organs. White blood cells, red blood cells and thrombocytes start to develop in the bone marrow. B-cells mature in the bone marrow, but T-cells mature in the thymus where they learn to recognise "objects" of the organism (Abbas et al., 2011). Matured immune cells encounter antigens, recognise or eliminate them in the secondary immune organs, e. g. lymph nodes, Peyers's patches, spleen or tonsils, see Fig. 5 (adopted and adjusted from (Delves [n. d.]).

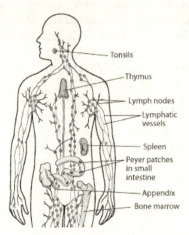

Fig. 5: Immune organs (adopted and adjusted from (Delves [n. d.]))

2.5   MECHANISMS OF THE NATURAL IMMUNE SYSTEM

Basic facts about fundamental mechanisms of the natural immune system are explained in the following subchapters. The emphasis is on the following mechanisms: mechanisms of tolerance, (non)-specific humoral and cell-mediated immune mechanisms.

2.5.1   IMMUNE TOLERANCE

Immune tolerance is the key mechanism of the NIS. Peripheral tolerance complements the central tolerance. It takes place in the tissue and nodules. It is maintained by apoptosis (physical elimination of the auto-reactive clones of the cells) or by an anergy (suppression of cells in case of their insufficient stimulation). Central tolerance is established in the bone marrow where positive selection (PS) and negative selection (NS) takes place (Murphy et al., 2008). The main aim of the positive selection is to eliminate non-functional receptors for B-cells and T-cells (de Castro and Timmis, 2002). The NIS eliminates B-cells and T-cells which do not react (or react very weakly) with self-antigens. B-cells or T-cells reacting more with self-antigens survive. The main aim of the negative selection is to eliminate auto-reactive lymphocytes (cells reacting against own cells). T-cells with strong affinity (strength of bind) for self-antigens presented by APC are eliminated by apoptosis (programmed cell death), (Abbas et al., 2011). Other T-cells survive and are differentiated towards mature T-cells. The negative selection process occurs in a similar manner as in case of T-cells. If these processes fail, some auto-reactive lymphocytes can escape. Two signal model of the B-cells activation is used for this purpose. The binding between the receptor of a B-cell (BCR) and the antigen is the first signal of activation (Murphy et al., 2008). This signal is not enough for the activation of the T-cell to take place, because the T-cell "has to have" information about the level of dangerousness of the antigen from various sources. T_h-cells are the messengers of the second (co-stimulation) signal. T_h-cell transmits the information about the antigens with the help of cytokines (communication molecules) towards B-cells and T-cells. If the lymphocytes do not receive the second signal on time, they can die by apoptosis or became anergic (immune unresponsiveness) and stay in the NIS (Sompayrac, 2012).

2.5.2 NON-SPECIFIC CELL-MEDIATED IMMUNE MECHANISMS

Phagocytosis is one of the most known non-specific immune mechanisms which are performed by phagocytic cells (e. g. macrophages, neutrophils, basophils, dendritic cells). These specialised cells engulf and ingest other cells or particles (e. g. harmful microorganisms, waste materials, non-functioning cells etc.) (Abbas and Lichtman, 2010). They use inner toxic products for elimination of danger "objects". Fig. 6 describes steps of phagocytic process:

- chemotaxis and adherence of microorganism to phagocyte,
- ingestion of the microorganism by phagocyte,
- formation of a phagosome,
- fusion of the phagosom with a lysosome containing digestive enzymes for degradation of the microorganism,
- digestion of ingested microorganism by enzymes,
- releasing of the waste material from the cell.

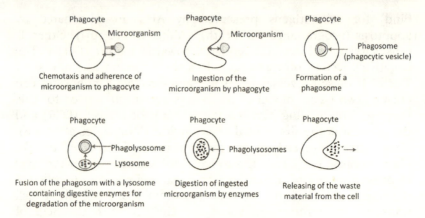

Fig. 6: Phagocytosis

2.5.3 NON-SPECIFIC HUMORAL IMMUNE MECHANISMS

An important regulator of the NIS, discovered by J. Bordet, is the complement system (Murphy et al., 2008), (Abbas et al., 2011). It is a collection of 30 – 40 proteins interacting with each other and with other objects of the NIS. A group of nine components (C_1 – C_9) is highly important and at first circulates in the blood circulation in a passive form. It can be activated by specific stimuli leading to the destruction of the plasmatic membrane of dangerous object by osmotic lysis process. Osmotic lysis is the final process of activation of a complement system where proteins of the complement system form into a shape which is able to sieve the membrane of the pathogen. Invasion of the structure of the antigenic membrane causes the catharsis of the membrane. Death of the pathogen is the result of the osmotic lysis.

2.5.4 SPECIFIC CELL-MEDIATED IMMUNE MECHANISMS

Specific cell-mediated immune processes encompass mechanisms of the T-cells. T-cells are white-blood cells which develop in the bone marrow and mature in the thymus. T-cells undergo positive selection in the thymus where T-cells with non-functional receptors (TCR) are eliminated. T-cells undergo negative selection also in the thymus where auto-reactive T-cells are destroyed. The crucial difference between B-cell and T-cell is the following: the most of T-cells are not able to bind to antigens directly, but only with the help of the APC presenting antigens with the MHC (HLA) molecules.

The most known types of T-cells are presented in the subchapter 2.2. Natural killer cells (NK) are very similar to the T_c-cells, because they have similar cytotoxic functions as T_c-cells. They are able to remove cancer cells or cells affected by a virus very quickly (Murphy et al., 2008), (Sompayrac, 2012).

2.5.5 SPECIFIC HUMORAL IMMUNE MECHANISMS

Another crucial specific humoral immune mechanism is the generation of antibodies. An antibody (Ab) is a molecule which is a part of the cytoplasmic membrane of the B-cell or moves in the blood stream in soluble form. It behaves as a receptor (surface structure – paratope) of the B-cell. It binds to the antigenic structures and recognises them. Physical and chemical properties enable them to initiate the binding process. Strength of binding is specified by the affinity. Higher affinity corresponds with stronger binding between antigen and the immune cell. Antibodies are produced by B-cells during humoral immune response. They have several functions (Murphy et al., 2008):

- neutralization of activities of toxins, viruses and other dangerous pathogens,
- opsonisation of pathogens (antibodies mark a pathogen for its ingestion and destruction),
- complement activation.

Clonal selection process is one of the most important humoral immune processes in the NIS, see Fig. 7. It was described by F. M. Burnet in 1959, and explains the process of generating antibodies. Mature naïve B-cells migrate from the bone marrow to the secondary lymphoid organs (e. g. lymph nodes) where they meet antigens. The B-cells can be stimulated by the antigenic peptides. The stimulation is caused by the binding process between the B-cell and the antigen. Immunocomplex antibody-antigen is developed after the recognition and stimulation process. It is the first activation signal for B-cells (Abbas and Lichtman, 2010). The second (confirmative) signal is necessary in order to avoid a dangerous or useless activation of the B-cell, see subchapter 2.5.1. Successful activation of the B-cell by the antigen leads to the clonal expansion where the B-cells proliferate and are differentiated into two forms: plasmatic cells producing antibodies and memory cells able to remember antigens from the past. Somatic mutation can contribute to the improvement of the affinity of the B-cell. Theory of the clonal selection explains the process of generating antibodies, but it does not explain the specificity of the antibodies. Heterogeneity of antibodies is the result of the gene segments recombination in chromosomes of the B-cells (Stites et al., 1994).

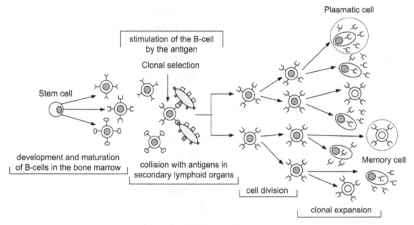

Fig. 7: Clonal selection

2.5.6   IDIOTYPIC NETWORK THEORY

Danish immunologist N. K. Jerne (Nobel prize winner in physiology or medicine) is the author of the idiotypic network theory (Jerne, 1974b). This theory supposes that the NIS is a dynamic system also in the cases when the B-cells or T-cells are not stimulated by common antigens. Immune response can be initiated by the existence of surface structures of pathogens – epitopes (antigenic determinants). Similar surface structures (idiotypes) occur also on B-cells. The surface structures of B-cells can also initiate an immune response if the NIS has never met with them before. The NIS initiates the production of further antibodies (anti-idiotypic antibodies) (de Castro and Timmis, 2002). The new surface structures of these new B-cells can also initiate the next immune response of the NIS. The anti-anti-idiotypic antibodies are produced again. The result of this process is a chain reaction. Internal image of the antigen is one of the most interesting aspects of the network theory. Chain reaction producing new antibodies causes that the

NIS has new antibodies useful for future attacks against non-self antigens. The antibodies can be inside the NIS before the attack, see Fig. 8 (adjusted from ((Husáková, 2009), Fig. 1b)). The B-cell B1 is able to recognise the epitope of the antigen and the idiotope of the B-cell B4. The NIS can evaluate the surface structures of the B-cell B4 as dangerous and initiate an immune reaction against the B-cell B4 – to produce the B-cells B2. The B-cell B2 can also have foreign surface fragments. The NIS can initiate the immune response with the production of the B-cells B3. Internal image of the antigen is depicted as the surface structure of the B-cell B4, because the immune cell was produced by the B-cell B1 as a response to the presence of the dangerous antigen. Its surface structure is similar to the surface structure of the antigen.

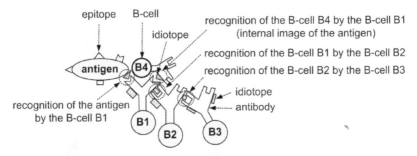

Fig. 8: Formation of the internal image of an antigen (adopted from (Dasgupta and Nino, 2008), Fig. 2.3), (adjusted from (Husáková, 2009), Fig. 1b)

3. ARTIFICIAL IMMUNE SYSTEMS

Artificial immune systems (AIS) can be perceived as systems able to represent and simulate behaviour of the natural immune system (NIS) allowing a more thorough analysis of the processes occurring on various levels of immunity. This is the computational immunology-based point of view that will be discussed in more detail in the chapter 4. A current definition of an artificial immune system can be found in the work of (de Castro and Timmis, 2002): *"Artificial immune systems (AIS) are adaptive systems, inspired by theoretical immunology and observed immune functions, principles and models, which are applied to problem solving."* The natural immune system is characterised by properties and mechanisms that have become an inspiration for problem solving not limited to the field of computer science. The main characteristics of the natural immune system that have drawn the attention of computer scientists are:

- Self-organisation and decentralisation: The natural immune system does not have a centre of organisation. It is an ambient system where everything is connected with everything. Immune cells are able to self-organise according to local interactions. These interactions give rise to a complex behaviour sustaining the organism in homeostasis. Self-organisation and decentralization are necessary for achieving a higher level of autonomy in the case of the artificial intelligence systems. For example, the theory of idiotypic network became the inspiration for the development of artificial immune network model where the components of this model (antibodies, lymphocytes) self-

organise in order to maintain homeostasis (Franzolini and
Olivier, 2009).

- Adaptation: Intelligent systems with adaptive mechanisms
  are able to be flexible and react faster. Adaptation and self-
  organisation are necessary for example in case of
  humanitarian or rescue operations where it is important to
  solve problems as fast as possible and often interact with
  each other. Symbrion is a robotic project that was aimed at
  the development of the self-organised system of
  autonomous robots (Kernbach et al., 2008). The structure
  of each robot is inspired by the structure of the lymph
  node. Autonomous robots are able to solve problems
  collectively. Obstacle avoidance is a typical example where a
  group of autonomous robots is able to unite to overcome
  obstacles. The group of autonomous robots thus behaves as
  a whole.

- Learning: The natural immune system learns from previous
  experience on the basis of a positive and a negative
  feedback received from the environment (de Castro and
  Timmis, 2002). The immune cells of the natural immune
  system have to be in touch with the possibly dangerous
  antigens. These antigens play the role of sources of
  learning. The immune cells "learn" the shapes of these
  antigens for faster reactions in the future. Learning is the
  key attribute of intelligent systems, because it helps with
  adaptation to the changing conditions of the environment
  in which the intelligent system occurs. Machine learning
  algorithms are developed and applied in data analysis.
  Group of artificial immune networks contains immunity-
  based algorithms used for data clustering (Timmis et al.,
  2000), (Leandro Nunes de and Fernando, 2002), (Li and
  Rong, 2009).

- Classification: The healthy natural immune system is able to
  distinguish self and non-self objects. Immune cells use
  surface receptors to detect these objects. Surface receptors
  play the role of detectors. The process of recognition
  becomes an inspiration for detecting anomalous signals in
  computer networks (Hofmeyr and Forrest, 1999). Various
  immunity-based algorithms are used to classify data into

groups in data analysis (Carter, 2000), (Goodman et al., 2002). Population-based algorithms are a group of immunity-based algorithms inspired by the (positive/negative/clonal) selection processes and are often used for classification (see Fig. 9).

- Self-repairing: Robustness of the natural immune system occurs if the organism is not in homeostasis, e. g. because of an infection. The natural immune system is able to function also in case of the disruption of homeostasis. Wide repertoire of immune cells and molecules is used to establish homeostasis. Robustness relates to the ability of the natural immune system to self-repair. The aim of the Autonomic Computing initiative is to develop auto-regulated systems able to autonomously self-configure, self-repair and self-optimise their behaviour (Müller, 2006). Autonomic computing paradigm is mainly inspired by the behaviour of human neural networks, but the immunity-based algorithms can be the inspiration of auto-regulated system development (Hart et al., 2007).

The natural immune system plays the role of an inspiration source in development of immune algorithms that can be used for various problems, e. g. for security of computational networks, in machine learning, data analysis, optimization tasks, planning or scheduling, see Fig. 9.

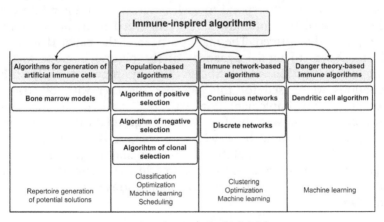

Fig. 9: Immune-inspired algorithms

The first ones to interconnect theoretical immunology with the computational intelligence were, in 1986, J. D. Farmer, N. H. Packard and A. S. Perelson (Farmer et al., 1986). They propose to represent immune cells and antigens as bit-strings of various lengths. The bit-string is composed of two values 0 and 1 (for simplicity) to represent amino acids which are contained in the surface structures of interacting objects, e. g. immune cells and antigens. In case of antibodies, antibody molecule is composed of a paratope (a part of the antibody for recognition the antigens) and an epitope (a part of the antibody which is used for recognition of different objects, e. g. pathogens). These two surface structures are represented as a collection (a list) of two values - 0 and 1, see Fig. 10 (adjusted from (Farmer et al., 1986)).

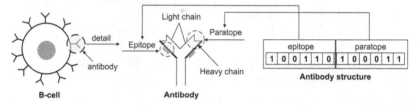

Fig. 10: Bit-string representation (adjusted from (Farmer et al., 1986))

These "data structures" have been used for mutual recognition of interacting objects – antibodies x antibodies and antibodies x antigens with the help of the Hamming distance measure. If the compared values correspond to each other, the bond is reinforced. The activity of the antibody is also reinforced if the antibody has recognised the antigen. The main purpose of the paper (Farmer et al., 1986) was to model dynamics of the natural immune system components within the artificial immune network. Differential equations were used for this purpose together with bit-strings. Computational implementation was not realised. It was only proposed, but it was the first work suggesting that the natural immune system could be viewed as a computational system. This model was later adjusted by H. Bersini and F. J. Varela. This adjustment was carried out in practice in the cart-pole balancing problem as one of the first practical applications of the AIS (Bersini and Varela, 1991).

Nowadays, four classes of immune algorithms exist, and each class is inspired by different aspect of the natural immune system. Bone marrow models are inspired by generation process of immune cells in the bone marrow (primary immune organ producing immune cells) (de Castro and Timmis, 2002). Bone marrow models use gene libraries and specific algorithms to generate potential solutions which are very close to an optimal solution. The bone marrow models are applied for example in the development of systems for detecting intrusions in computer networks (Hofmeyr and Forrest, 2000) or in job shop scheduling problem (Coello et al., 2003). Population-based immune algorithms are the second class of immune algorithms. This group contains three key representatives: algorithm of positive selection, algorithm of negative selection and clonal selection-based immune algorithm. The first two algorithms are inspired by the immune processes accepting only functional and desirable immune cells able to fight effectively with danger objects. Clonal selection-based immune algorithm is based on the clonal selection principle that is responsible for generation of the new immune cells able to recognise objects potentially dangerous for the organism. Algorithm of positive and negative selection is mainly used for classification and recognition tasks. Typical example here is the application in anomalies detection in computer networks (Hofmeyr and Forrest, 1999) or scheduling problems at a university (Malim et al., 2006). Clonal selection algorithm is applied for optimization purposes (de Castro and Von Zuben, 2000) or in prediction of protein structures (Cutello et al., 2007). Idiotypic network theory became the inspiration for artificial immune networks. This theory expects the continuation of the activity of the natural immune system also without the presence of antigens – objects able to initiate the natural immune system. This group of algorithms is applied in modelling and simulation of the NIS (continuous artificial immune networks), movement of mobile robots (Ichikawa et al., 1998), recognition of DNA sequences (Hunt and Cooke, 1996), cluster analysis (Timmis and Neal, 2001) or classification problems (Secker et al., 2003) (discrete artificial immune networks). The dendritic cell algorithm is the last representative of immunity algorithms. Dendritic cells are the source of inspiration for this class of algorithms. They play various roles, functioning as messengers for different immune cells or supporting their stimulation or differentiation. Machine learning is an example of their application domain (Greensmith et al., 2005), (Greensmith et al., 2010).

Immunity-based algorithms have been successfully applied in solving different problems, but some researchers claim that this direction of research is in a "dead end", because the majority of immunity-based algorithms are based on simplified views of the processes occurring in the NIS (Stepney et al., 2004), (Timmis, 2006), (Timmis, 2007). Adaptive layer of the NIS is the main source of inspiration for most of these algorithms. Innate layer of the NIS is less complex in comparison to the adaptive immunity and has also very interesting features which can be used in the development of novel immunity-inspired solutions (Twycross and Aickelin, 2007). Dendritic cell algorithm is one of the first steps in the development of an innate immunity-based algorithm, because it is inspired by dendritic cells existing between innate and adaptive immunity. It is obvious that the NIS cannot be represented as a closed system and separated from the surrounding parts of the organism. The NIS is an ambient system. It cooperates with the adjacent complex systems – the nervous system, the endocrine system and the reproductive system. Current immunity-based algorithms suppose the NIS is closed system, i. e. it does not cooperate with other biological (sub)systems. Future research in the AIS field must thus focus on the following (de Castro and Timmis, 2002), (Castro and Timmis, 2003):

- to develop of a new immunity-inspired algorithms for specific problems,
- to find "killer-application" for which the immunity-based algorithms can be applied as the best solution,
- to improve already developed immunity-based algorithms,
- to use the immunity-based algorithms in new application areas,
- to analyse in detail the immunity-based algorithms (ways of application of the algorithms together with methods of representation, development and implementation).

Immunity-based algorithms are perceived as an alternative approach for solving problems similar to those that can be solved using the artificial neural networks or genetic algorithms.

4. Computational Immunology

Biology and medicine constitute the areas of interest for computational biology, bioinformatics and computational systems biology. These three research fields overlap, and it is difficult to find a clear definition that would be able to differentiate between them. Bioinformatics focuses mainly on the development of software tools for acquiring, storing, organising, analysing and visualising bio(medical) data (Huerta et al., 2000), (Nair, 2007). Computational biology tends to use already existing or new theoretical methods and approaches (e. g. mathematical modelling, artificial or computational intelligence) in the study of biological systems. Computational systems biology is an approach using systems theory for the study of emergence phenomena occurring on a varied levels in biological systems (Likic et al., 2010). A common attribute of these three areas of research is an attempt to understand processes occurring in biological systems with the aim to predict their behaviour with changes of various parameters, and to develop effective drugs. The following subchapters introduce the subarea of computational biology – computational immunology, and present it from the point of view of the initial research attempts, the most common modelling approaches and future perspectives.

4.1 Introduction to computational immunology

The NIS is studied not only for the possibility to develop efficient immunity-based algorithms. In applying its methods and techniques, computational immunology uncovers the amazing world and complexity underlying the natural immune system. It interconnects elements of biology, medicine, chemistry, immunology, modelling, simulation, mathematics, physics, statistics and computer science (artificial or computational intelligence) together with social awareness that is necessary for efficient communication with experts, see Fig. 11. Computational immunology (CI) is a specific subarea of computational biology concentrating on the inner life of the NIS in order to discover efficient strategies which could be used to influence the behaviour of the NIS.

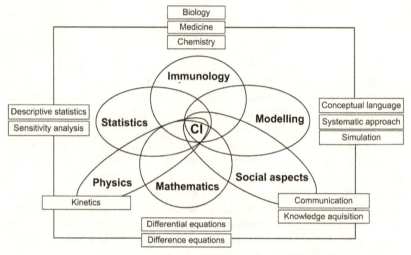

Fig. 11: Interdisciplinarity of computational immunology

4.1.1   IMMUNE NETWORKS AT THE BEGINNING

Continuous immune networks represent the first attempt at modelling of some specific aspects of the NIS. The origins of the CI date to 1974 when Nobel prize winner N. K. Jerne proposed the idiotypic network theory explaining the possible activation of the NIS without the presence of dangerous antigens (Jerne, 1974b). The NIS can be stimulated also by molecules which are on the surface of antibody molecules. These can be detected as antigens by the NIS. In his paper (Jerne, 1974b), Jerne mainly concentrates on the philosophical aspects of idiotypic network behaviour. In the same year, he observed the dynamic behaviour of lymphocytes and antibodies without pathogens. Interactions between these "immune objects" lead the formation of an immune network (Jerne, 1974a). Differential equations were used to model the dynamics of this network.

4.1.2 CONCEPT OF SHAPE SPACE

The concept of shape space was proposed by A. S. Perelson and G. F. Oster in 1979, for quantitative representation of components in the NIS (Perelson and Oster, 1979). This concept is based on the binding process between immune cells and antigens using the complementarity principle. Interacting objects behave like keys and locks. The immune cell "tries to find" an appropriate key (antigen). Affinity (non-negative value) represents the strength of binding between objects. Each object is a point in the system of coordinates. Affinity radius (threshold) surrounds this point and represents the ability to recognise the objects. Larger affinity radius leads to a higher probability of interaction with objects, see Fig. 12.

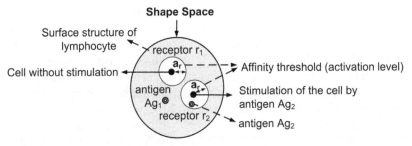

Fig. 12: Shape space

Objects are predestined to be represented in the shape space by the application domain. Anything from packets which are transferred through the computational network, to users specifying preferences for movies, artificial agents with abilities to solve specific problem or breeds of dogs and their properties, can constitute points of the shape space. Objects and their properties are mainly represented as binary strings, first proposed in the volume (Farmer et al., 1986) for use in computational immunology. The type of shape space used is determined by the data type that is applied for properties of objects representation. The shape spaces according to (de Castro and Timmis, 2002) are:

- Real-valued shape space: shape space with vectors of real values,
- Integer-valued shape space: shape space with vectors of integer values,
- Hamming shape space: vector of symbols from finite alphabet or binary strings,
- Symbolic shape space: vector of different types of strings where at least one of them is symbolic.

4.1.3 THE FIRST COMPUTATIONAL MODEL OF THE NATURAL IMMUNE SYSTEM

The first computational model of the NIS was presented in 1992 by F. Celada and P. E. Seiden (Celada and Seiden, 1992). The model is based on the cellular automata (CA) – mathematical and dynamical models able to model and simulate complex biological processes with cells following simple local rules. The CA model uses N-dimensional matrix (1D, 2D, 3D). Each element of the matrix is a cell. The state of the CA is based on the states of the cells in the matrix. CA evolves in discrete time steps with the same deterministic rules. The state of the cell changes on the basis of its own state and state of the cells which are around it. The CA-based model of Celada and Seiden contains immune cells (B-cells, T-cells, antigens, APC with surface structures (antibodies, MHC) which were represented as binary strings with the length of 8 bits. Representation of B-cells and T-cells together with surface structures is presented in Fig. 13 (adopted from ((Beauchemin, 2002), Fig. 3)). Each surface structure is represented by binary strings, and interactions between cells are represented as XOR operation – only complementary structures can interact with each other. CA represents key interactions related to the initiation and regulation of humoral immune response. CA considers the strength of interactions between cells. The strength is modelled and based on probability rules. Deterministic rules are not applied in this case. The state of the cell is changed according to the cells which interact with the cell in the same position. Mobility of cells in the CA is considered. The model is perceived as the initial study for whole a family of IMMSIM models - bit-strings-based CA. Programming code of the IMMSIM model is presented in (Celada and Seiden, 1992). Selected members of the IMMSIM family are introduced in the subchapter 4.2.2.

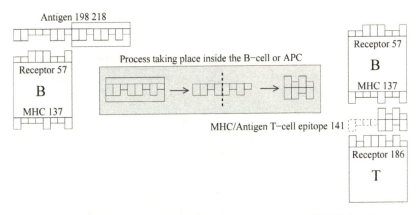

Fig. 13: Surface structures of B-cells and T-cells in IMMSIM model (adopted from (Beauchemin, 2002), Fig. 3)

4.2 APPROACHES

The progress in the field of computational immunology can be traced through conferences or journal papers, books, case studies and projects focusing on individual topics related to the scale of organisation (molecular, cellular, tissue, organ or organism) in a biological system. Research topics use specific approaches (equation-based models, cellular automata, Petri nets, etc.), and the final results are presented in the form of conceptual, mathematical or software solutions, see Fig. 14. The following subchapters will look at the progress in the CI according to levels of organisation in a biological system. Selected studies mentioned here have contributed significantly to the understanding of the innate or adaptive immunity.

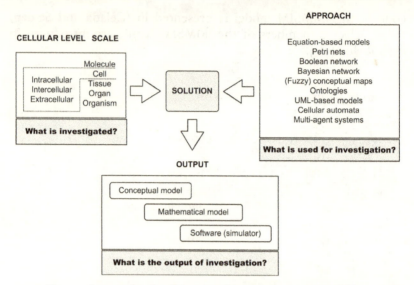

Fig. 14: Approaches for the natural immune system modelling

4.2.1 Processes studied on the molecular scale

Biological networks (signalling, gene regulatory or metabolic) are in the centre of interest of mathematicians and computational scientists, especially because of their complexity. This complexity is caused by the amount of components and interactions between them, and possible feedback loops which contribute to the difficulty to study them directly in the organism. The quantitative approaches that can be used for the analysis of biological networks are differential equations, Petri nets and agent-based systems.

Differential equations focus on models of interactions occurring on the global level of the investigated system. They are used for studying changes in the concentrations of components in the biological systems per time unit. They are very useful for modelling different biological pathways, since they do not consider properties and behaviour of all the individual entities of the system. Simulation with differential equations means to solve equations. Complexity of the system determines the number of equations needed. This is the main drawback of these equation-based models because their complexity limits the scope of their usage. It is often necessary to carry out a large amount of simplification in order to obtain a suitable model. Ordinary differential equations (ODE) are used for modelling control mechanisms of the JAK (Janus kinase)-STAT (Signal transducer and activator of transcription) signal transduction pathway which is responsible for example for innate and adaptive immunity control, cell growth or apoptosis regulation (Yamada et al., 2003). Smolen (SMOLEN et al., 2003) describes the process of the change in concentration of Ca_2+ ion able to transmitting intracellular messages within the cell. The process is modelled with the ODE.

Petri nets are formal mathematical models representing distributed systems. They can be used also for modelling of biological phenomena. One of the first applications in biology domain is mentioned in (Reddy et al., 1993) where Petri nets are used in modelling of metabolic processes. Petri nets were also used for the development of discrete model of signal transduction pathway (mating pheromone response) of one species of yeast – Sacchromyces cerevisiae (Sackmann et al., 2006). Metabolic signalling pathways, pathways of signal transduction or gene regulatory networks can be modelled also with Petri nets, see more details e. g. in (Pinney et al., 2003), (Hardy and Robillard, 2004) or (Painter, 2009).

Multi-agent-based systems (MAS) are stochastic systems consisting of entities called agents able to solve specific problems without an intervention from humans. They interact (communicate, coordinate, cooperate) with each other to achieve the required goal or to compete with each other, such as in the case of limited sources. They are not often used for modelling processes on the molecular level, but have several other applications (especially frameworks or conceptual solutions). NK-kB intracellular signalling pathway was analysed using agent-based approach in (Pogson et al., 2008). This pathway is crucial for regulation of the immune response. NK-kB is the transcription factor influencing the expression of specific genes which are necessary for inflammatory response, cell growth or cell death. Activation of this pathway is strictly regulated. Some diseases (e. g. cancer, arthritis, asthma) can occur if the pathway is damaged. Each agent (transcription factor, receptor) is represented by Communicating stream X-Machine – computational model similar to the finite state automaton including memory and ability to send messages. This model can be used for the study of different properties of the signalling pathway, for example the impacts of changes on the level of proteins in different phases of signalling pathway regulation. X-Machines are used not only for molecular species representation, but also for modelling of cells, see (Coakley et al., 2006). Agent-based approach is applied for blackboard-based architecture Cellulat focusing on modelling of intracellular signalling pathways (Pérez et al., 2002). Originally, the blackboard architecture is proposed for sharing information between more expert agents during problem solving. It plays the role of the internal communication structure of the cell where two main agents are distinguished. Internal agents represent components of intracellular network (e. g. proteins, enzymes) interacting with each other. Interface agents mediate contact between outer and inner environment of the cell. They represent the surface receptors of the cell, and are responsible for secretion of signalling molecules. Intracellular signals are registered by the blackboard as events which can activate/deactivate internal agents. The Ca2+ signalling pathway is modelled with Cellulat as a case study. Cellulat was conceptually proposed in (Pérez et al., 2002) as the method for modelling of cognitive abilities (learning, memory, pattern recognition) of internal agents (proteins, enzymes) and high-level space organisation of signalling pathways. Java-based framework DECAF (Distributed Environment Centered Agent Framework) is based on multi-agent systems and used for modelling of biological networks, i. e. MAP kinase pathway (mitogen-activated protein kinases) (Khan et al., 2003). This framework uses the species-as-agent paradigm, where a group of similar entities of the pathway is represented as one agent (one class) because of the amount of components in the system. The movement of molecules is directed by the Brownian motion. The results of the simulation of this pathway were compared with the results mentioned in different papers using differential equations instead of multi-agent systems (Schoeberl et al., 2002). A platform for simulation of biological networks is proposed e. g. in (Ren et al., 2008). Functionalities of the platform are described for a model representing the protein network. The structure of the platform is multi-layered thus integrating bio-entities represented as autonomous agents (e. g. parts of the DNA molecule, proteins, cells). Each component of the network has a collection of attributes, methods of behaviour, mechanisms of communication and functional information (abilities of the entity and how they can be used). Bio-entities interact with each other and form a society developing gradually into a network shape. Bio-entities migrate, replicate, reproduce (with mutation and crossover) and communicate. ACL (Agent Communication Language) and XML-based communication language (bio-network communication language) is proposed in the platform.

4.2.2 PROCESSES STUDIED ON THE CELLULAR SCALE

Cellular automata (CA) and multi-agent systems (MAS) are the most suitable methods for modelling of interactions occurring on the cellular level of the organism, because they focus on attributes and behaviour of individual components of the system. They model complex interactions which can lead to an aggregate behaviour, and emergent phenomena which are visible on the global level of the investigated system.

Various CA-based simulators of immune processes have been developed in the attempt to answer questions about the influence of pathogens on the homeostasis in the NIS. The first computational model of the NIS called IMMSIM has been already mentioned in the subchapter 4.1.3. This model has laid the foundations for further IMMSIM-based models of the NIS. An extension of the original IMMSIM model – IMMSIM3 is proposed in (Bezzi and Cellada, 1997). It integrates processes of humoral and cellular immunity. This model looks at cytotoxic T-cells, viruses, interleukins and interferons. M. Meier-Schellersheim and G. Mack from the University of Hamburg published the SIMMUNE model using a 3D lattice for modelling of different compartments of the NIS, e. g. lymphoid vessel or thymus (Meier-Schellersheim and Mack, 1999). Cells are perceived as units able to process signals and information. Signal is composed of molecules binding to the surface receptors of the cell. The cells make decisions based on the cellular stimulus response mechanism using a set of conditional actions (rules). SIMMUNE software is composed of SIMMUNE Modeller (visual interface for setting interactions between cells), SIMMUNE Cell Designer (designer for morphology of the cell) and SIMMUNE simulator (simulator of interactions). 3D stochastic CA was used for the next version of IMMSIM - C-IMMSIM. This version was developed by F. Castiglione. It integrates helper T-cells, cytotoxic T-cells, B-cells producing antibodies, dendritic cells and macrophages. These cells interact with each other according to a set of rules. This model considers the areas of antigens presentation, MHC restriction, cooperation between cells, maturation of immune response, immune memory, clonal selection, chemotaxis, education process of T-cell in thymus, hypermutation of antibodies, danger signals and idiotypic network. More details can be found for example in (Rapin et al., 2010). The C-IMMSIM version was used for modelling of the infection of the Epstein-Barr virus (Castiglione et al., 2007). A parallel version of IMMSIM - ParIMM covering humoral and cellular immune processes is proposed in (Bernaschi and Castiglione, 2001). Cellular automata have also been used to examine the dynamics of infection caused by HIV virus (Zorzenon dos Santos and Coutinho, 2001). This model tries to model basic phases of the infection which are observed in the organism. It looks at interactions between HIV virus, CD4+ T-cells and monocytes. Cellular automata-based simulator of HIV-I virus infection was developed for the study of the role of mediators (especially IL-1, IL-5) in regulation activities of the NIS. The influence of the HIV virus on the helper T-cells and B-cells, and the dynamics of two classes of helper T-cells (Th1 and Th2) during infection have also been examined. In order to model the behaviour of the cell in CA, rules in combination with genetic-based approach have been applied here. Genes of chromosomes represent rules. Genetic operators use the genetic information (rules) for triggerring specific reactions of the cell of CA (Grilo et al., 2002).

CA have some limitations, especially in the movement of cells, the representation of communication and the complex interactions between them. The MAS is a more efficient approach since it can represent the analysed system in more details. Reactions of the NIS to the presence of a virus are modelled with the agent-based approach in a 3D environment Breve (Jacob et al., 2004). Antibodies production is observed during the primary and the secondary immune response. Interactions between tissue cells, viruses, B-cells, helper T-cells, killer T-cells or macrophages are represented.

Agent-based approach is used for the study of a serious infectious disease called Experimental Visceral Leishmaniasis (EVL) (Flugge et al., 2009). This disease is caused by an intracellular parasite of the genus Leishmania. It is spread through sand-flies of the genus Phlebotomus in the Old World, and of the genus Lutzomyia in the New World. Granuloma formation is the key process of the course of this disease, and it is not yet fully understood. It is not clear whether a positive or a negative role is played by the microenvironment (where the granulomas are formed). Domain and computational model of a small fragment of the liver and a granuloma formation has been developed, according to the CoSMoS process that can be used for complex systems modelling and simulation (Andrews et al., 2010). The study does not attempt to develop a complete and plausible model, but aims to support communication among experts and computer scientists with the aid of the 3D visualisation. Tissue-scale agent-based model analysing the dynamics of NK-T cells and Kuppfer cells during the initial phases of granuloma formation is developed as a continuation study of EVL (Moore et al., 2013). A complex autoimmune disease called Experimental autoimmune encephalomyelitis (EAE) has also been examined with the help of the agent-based approach (Greaves et al., 2012), (Williams et al., 2013). The EAE is caused by the decomposition of myelin material covering the axons of neural cells. Simulator ARTIMMUS (Artificial Murine Multiple Sclerosis Simulation) which is developed by M. Read, offers the environment for experimentation, for example for an investigation of the interactions between receptors of dendritic cells and T-cells (T_h-cells and T_{reg}-cells) which play a key role in this disease (Greaves et al., 2012), (Williams et al., 2013). Agent systems can also be applied in modelling of Peyer's patches - organised lymphoid tissues responsible for eliminating antigens in the small intestine (Alden et al., 2012), (Alden, 2012). The model analyses the organogenesis of this complex biological system as it is not obvious why the patches vary in quantity and size, or why they are formed in different locations of the small intestine. The simulator PPSim has been developed for organogenesis visualisation. Spartan (Simulation parameter analysis R toolkit application) has been developed and is used for data analysis of in silico results of simulations (Alden et al., 2013). Lymph nodes are similar to the Peyer's patches filtering the lymph. Humoral immune response is analysed in the presence of antigens in the lymph node (Belkacem and Foundil, 2012). Various immune cells and processes are involved in obtaining statistical information about the amount of immune cells in different locations of lymph node during infection. AnyLogic has been used for development of agent-based models of this complex system where behaviour of immune cells is represented by state diagrams.

4.2.3 Processes studied on the tissue scale

Tissue is a complex system composed of many autonomous components – cells. Several methods can be applied in the study of the complexity of this system. This system may be described as a collection of Partial differential equations (PDE), and the processes occurring on the global level are examined by this method. The PDE represent the basis of a continuous model developed to describe movements within heterogeneous tissue composed of different cell subpopulations (Painter, 2009). PDE can be used also in cancer modelling, such as in tumor growth modelling in healthy tissues. Mathematical models of tumor invasion based on the PDE and ODE are proposed in (McGillen et al., 2012). Here, the attention is focused on a better understanding of the tumour acidity and its invasion. A mathematical model of cancer cell invasion has been developed with the help of PDE, looking at interactions between cancer cells and host tissue, i. e. adhesion of cells and adhesion in the view of cell-extracellular matrix (Chaplain et al., 2011). Processes taking place on the local level, i. e. between individual components of the system are not taken into consideration here.

CA-based model of tumor tissue development using the square lattice structure is proposed in (Takayanagi et al., 2006). Interactions between cytotoxic T-cells and tumor cells are modelled with the influence of communication molecules – cytokines. The main purpose of the model is to investigate how cytotoxic T-cells interact with tumor tissue. Tumour induced angiogenesis is modelled in (Topa, 2006) with the help of CA where changes in cancer tissues and their neighbours are analysed with the use of a graph of CA – thus combining the CA with graph-based theory.

Agent-based systems can represent collective and aggregate behaviour with complex interactions occurring during tissue structure formation. MAS architecture is proposed for modelling tissues on the cell level in (Santos et al., 2004) who perceives the tissue as an interconnected discrete non-linear dynamic system with many decision-making autonomous agents. The behaviour of various types of tissue is the product of the combination of interactions between cells and cells with extracellular matrix behaving as a scaffold for the movement of cells. Environmental context is the main global data structure managing all information about cell agents, tissue agents (collection of cell agents) and the environment. It monitors states of the whole tissue system and plays a role of a map showing the actual state of the tissue. The various states of cell agents are modelled with finite state machines and the following processes of cell agents are considered: movement, death, mitosis or exchange of chemical substances between cells. The main aim of the proposed architecture is the modelling of the self-organisation principles. The purpose of the Epitheliome project is to develop a model of functional epithelium (Walker et al., 2004), (Smallwood and Holcombe, 2006). Agent-based method is used in the development of this biological system, since the formation of epithelium is an emergent property of the system composed of many cells. Cell cycle is modelled in the initial studies on the basis of information received in vitro. This model comprises stem cells, transit amplifying cells, (post)mitotic cells and dead cells. The study aims to provide a model of the normal behaviour of epithelium, and to investigate possible anomalies in this behaviour which could lead to the pathologies.

4.3   PERSPECTIVES

Many research teams and laboratories have been established and are involved in the study of the natural immune system. It is not possible for this monograph to include them all, just as it is not possible to mention all research papers, books or projects related to the computational immunology. One successful past project and one current initiative is going to be reviewed here as representative of the ideas already put to practice as well as the directions for future research. The project ImmunoGrid (The European Virtual Human Immune System Project), one of the best known and most successful projects, got underway in 2006 with the financial support from the European commission. The main aim of this project was to develop the simulator of human immune system that would be able to offer a clear image of the processes occurring on the molecular, cellular or organ levels with the help of grid technologies. A further aim was to support vaccine development, and optimization of immune therapies. This project resulted in various simulators, for example the simulator analysing the influence of different viruses (influenza, HIV or Epstein-Barr). The ImmunoComplexiT initiative was initiated in 2011 with the objective to better understand and model complexity of the NIS on molecular, cellular and organ scale of organisation with respect to time and space. Mathematical, statistical, philosophical and computer science-based methods should contribute to the overall understanding of the NIS. The result of this initiative has been the network of 15 interdisciplinary national and international teams who cooperate together to address the main future challenges as specified in (Lavelle et al., 2012):

- objective identification of immune system cell populations,
- lymphocyte population dynamics and repertoire selection: integration of multilevel/multi-scale data and dynamic modelling,
- understanding resilience or instabilities of perturbations, immune dysfunctions in order to improve immuno-intervention strategies,
- extract, visualise and organise immunological knowledge from specialist immunological literature,
- contribute to global evaluation of complex systems and risk issue.

Current research in the field of the computational immunology focuses on the search and analysis of effective and computationally undemanding solutions which could help in the development of plausible models. In the case of models development, it is necessary to support validity of results obtained during simulation. It is not acceptable to infer final conclusions about behaviour of the analysed system only on the basis of visual interpretation of simulation outputs. Different statistical methods (techniques of sensitivity analysis) help to examine the influence of changes in parameter values on the behaviour of the system. These results can be compared with the behaviour of the real system. Experts can play a part in determining the validity of the model by ascertaining whether the behaviour of the artificial biological system under specific conditions is the same/similar or different in comparison to the natural biological system. Current research in modelling of the

NIS focuses also on combining different modelling approaches for the development of hybrid systems (Grilo et al., 2002), (Guo and Tay, 2007), (Banerjee and Moses, 2009), (Kim and Lee, 2012). Since the multiple scales of organisation present in the NIS cannot all be modelled using the same method. Another approach to this problem was to make use of methods originally developed for different practical purposes. For example, holonic systems were firstly introduced in 1967 by the Hungarian philosopher A. Koestler in (Koestler, 1967). He defined a holon as a self-similar structure occurring in biological and social systems. Holon is a building block with a hierarchical and recursive structure. It is a part of a bigger structure and is composed of self-similar components which also have components. Agents are similar to holons, but they do not consist of parts having the same or similar structure. Holonic systems were mainly proposed for real-time processes occurring in a relatively stable environment where predefined rules have to be fulfilled and no innovative or random processes occur. Holonic systems are used mainly in industrial systems and production. Holonic principles offer themselves as a solution for problems where many different scales of organisation exist. Cancer is a complex disease involving the molecular, cellular, tissue and organ scale. The use of holonic architecture in cancer research is advocated in (Masoudi-Nejad and Meshkin, 2014). The motivation and overall goal of computational biology (immunology) is the same for all researchers and their teams – to improve the quality of human life not only through medical treatment, but also through the use of computer science, mathematics, data analysis and engineering. Computational immunology research is difficult, time consuming, but exciting. Some difficulties that can be encountered have already been mentioned, but it does not mean that problems cannot be solved. It is necessary to find suitable and efficient "weapons" or their combinations for dealing with diseases in order to re-establish homeostasis which will increase the quality of our lives.

5. EXPLORATION OF IMMUNITY – CoSMoS-based Approach

Investigation of complex systems requires systematic approach. CoSMoS (Complex Systems Modelling and Simulation) is the approach offering guidelines for systematic study of complex systems phenomena. It is the process and infrastructure that is used for exploration of complex systems with modelling and simulation. It has been proposed within the CoSMoS project whose aim was to support analysis, design, development and validation of models dealing with complex systems (Andrews et al., 2011). Development of CoSMoS process is based on different case studies for verification the presence of all necessary components of CoSMoS process (Read et al., 2009), (Andrews et al., 2010), (Andrews et al., 2011), (Alden, 2012). CoSMoS process is structured into the three phases. Each phase, except the last one, is divided into products defining the content and output of each phase, see Fig. 15 (Andrews et al., 2010):

1. Discovery phase: Application domain, research questions and hypotheses are determined. The following activities are distinguished in this phase: domain modelling, scoping and documenting. The phase contains these products:
    a. Research context defines the scope and the purpose of the CoSMoS project. Research questions and hypotheses (related to the application domain) are specified together with technical and human

limitations. Information sources used in the next products are also mentioned.

b. Domain model is mainly a collection of conceptual models. These models represent information about domain of interest into the form of informal sketches or detailed pictures, graphs or diagrams. Information caught in this way helps to ease the communication between domain modeller and expert. Expected behaviour diagram (EBD) should be the first step in visualisation of observed behaviour in complex system.

2. Development phase: Simulation platform is developed in this phase. The following activities are distinguished in this phase: platform implementation, scoping, interacting, modelling and experimenting. The phase contains the following products:

a. Platform model adjusts the domain model for its implementation into the programming code. Abstraction is often necessary for facilitation development of this code. Modelling approaches (e. g. MAS, CA, (ordinary, partial) differential equations (DE)) and development tools (e. g. NetLogo, AnyLogic, Repast, Breve), that are going to be used, are also mentioned in this phase. Emergent phenomena are removed in this phase in comparison to the domain model because these processes should appear spontaneously during simulation.

b. Simulation platform deals with the implementation of the platform model into the executable code. Testing of simulation platform is a necessary part for ensuring reliability and correctness of the computational model.

3. Exploration phase: This phase focuses on simulation and analysis of results which were received from these simulations.

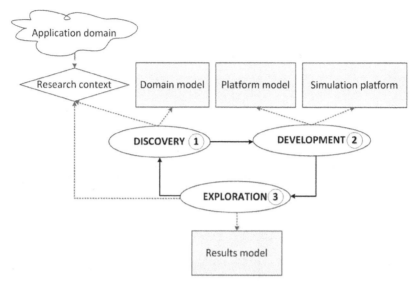

Fig. 15: CoSMos process

CoSMoS framework is successfully applied in development of models dealing with processes occurring in the natural immune systems. The CoSMoS is applied in the investigation of the autoimmune disease - experimental autoimmune encephalomyelitis (murine model of multiple sclerosis) (Read et al., 2009) or for simulations of lymphoid tissue (Peyer's patches) formation (Alden, 2012). Model of prostate cell division and differentiation is built with the usage of Petri nets and the CoSMoS process (Droop et al., 2011). Model and simulation of granuloma formation in infectious disease visceral leishmaniasis (kala-azar) is realised also on the basis of CoSMoS process (Flugge et al., 2009). This framework is partially applied for the investigation and conceptual modelling of processes occurring in the lymph node of the mouse, see the chapter 8.

6. CONCEPTUAL MODELLING IN COMPUTATIONAL IMMUNOLOGY

Conceptual modelling is mainly mentioned in software or knowledge engineering together with simulation. Conceptualisation is the process of the identification of the most important concepts (real or unreal things, feelings, processes, characteristics, etc.) and relations between them of the application domain that is in the centre of our interest. Conceptualisation is useful for improvement of communication between people during problem solving, decision making, learning or teaching. It is the iterative process during which we try to find convenient abstraction level. (Nance, 1994) distinguishes conceptual model and communicative model. Conceptual model exists only in the human mind in the form of the mental model. Communicative model is an explicit expression of the conceptual model, e. g. in the graph structure, diagram, ontology, etc. (Lacy et al., 2001) distinguishes domain-oriented model including detailed information about modelled application domain. Design-oriented model is adjusted domain model for the usage in the software development or simulations. The similar classification appears also in the CoSMoS process where the domain model is created during the discovery phase. Design-oriented model has similar usage as the platform model in the CoSMoS. Domain model is modified for its implementation into the programming code. The widely accepted definition of the conceptual model does not exist, but common characteristics can be identified: simplification of the reality (abstraction), iterative development, independence of any programming language or programming paradigm, see the chapter 5. Fig. 16 depicts relations between models that can be created before the outputs of simulation are analysed. "A modeller" investigates an area of interest and constructs a mind-based implicit model containing the most important facts (concepts and relations between them) about investigated problem. These concepts are visually depicted in the explicit model that is used for discusses about application domain. It plays the role of the source material for specification of an executable model containing programming code that is used for simulation purposes. The following subchapters introduce various approaches used in conceptual modelling in computational immunology.

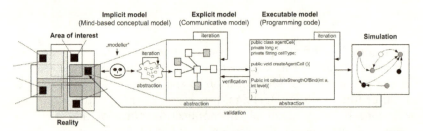

Fig. 16: Conceptual modelling

6.1   Concept maps

Concept map is a structure used for representation and organisation of information and relations between them in visual manner. This informal approach was proposed by J. D. Novak in his research program at the Cornell University in 1972 (Novak and Cañas, 2006). The research program was focused on understanding how the children learn, i. e. how the knowledge is changed during their study. Concept mapping is based on the learning psychology proposed by D. Ausubel (Ausubel, 1963): *"If I had to reduce all of educational psychology to just one principle I would say this: The most important single factor influencing learning is what the learner already knows. Ascertain this and teach him accordingly."* The meaningful learning theory of D. Ausubel claims that learning process and understanding of new knowledge is mainly based on the idea what person already knows about the studied topic. The actual understanding of specific problem is extended on the basis of previous experience, information and knowledge. Concept maps have very simple structure - only two key elements are necessary for concept maps building: concept and linking word. The concept represents entity (a class, an object, a process, a property) of the investigated application domain. Linking word represents relationship between concepts of the same or different domains (cross-links). Linking words specify context that is used for comprehension of concepts meaning. Fig. 17 depicts basic elements of concept maps.

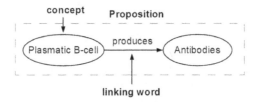

Fig. 17: Key elements of the concept map

Concept maps are powerful tool for generation of new ideas, knowledge and communicate them during brainstorming in problem solving and decision making. They help students during learning to understand complex topics, because the complexity can be visualised by the concept map. Concept maps are also useful for teachers, because they are able to identify valid and invalid sequences of knowledge by comparing concept map of learner and teacher. Concept maps can capture tacit knowledge of experts that are integrated into the knowledge-based system (e. g. expert system).

There is not pre-defined sequence of steps for concept maps development. General approach is mentioned e. g. in (Novak, 1990), (Novak, 2002) or (Novak and Cañas, 2006). Firstly, it has to be obvious why a concept map is developed and which application domain is going to be mapped. Core concepts of application domain are identified after that. These concepts can be ordered according to the priority or generality in the table(s). Preliminary concept map is built on the basis of these table(s) on the paper or the specific software tool can be used, e. g. CmapTools, VUE,

LucidChart, SmartDraw, OpenOffice Draw, etc. Concept map is revised after that, because new concepts or relations between them can appear, change their position or can be deleted because of their uselessness. Relations between concepts of different domains (cross-links) can be represented after concept map revision, but the purpose of the concept map building answer the question if the cross-links are necessary. Revision of the concept map should be done again - re-positioning of concepts, linking-words or cross-links can improve the overall clarity of the concept map.

Concept maps can add value also into understanding of the natural immune system behaviour. The following subchapters describe development of the topic maps-based information and knowledge structure - concept map ComImmuno-AIS for uncovering relations between immunology, computational immunology and immunological computations, because it need not to be obvious where the differences exist and how these three research areas are connected (Husáková, 2015c). The topic map should help with the orientation in these three areas without reading a lot of study materials.

6.1.1 Development of the concept map

Concept maps are highly individual. Individuality of concept maps is caused by various learning styles, different learning preconditions, diverse experience or emotions playing key role in learning process. It means that if the concept maps are developed for the one application domain, the output of their authors are mostly different. Each one has different notion about the reality. Development of the concept map ComImmuno-AIS is divided into the following steps (Husáková, 2015c):

1. Preparation phase: This phase mentions purpose of the concept map, information sources used for concept map development, keywords emphasizing topics covered by the concept map and approach for concept mapping (paper-based, software support).

2. Domain of interest: Description of the application domain(s) can clarify some parts of the concept map or highlight its key parts.

3. Backbone of the concept map: Crucial concepts are identified with limited collection of linking-words. They are

ordered in tables and visualised in the VUE environment, see Fig. 18.

4. Backbone extension: The main attention is paid to the concept map extension with concepts and linking-words for each application domain without cross-links.

5. Refinement: Correctness of information and knowledge is checked. The help of an expert is useful, especially in case of multi-disciplinary concept map development.

6. Backbone extension with cross-links: Cross-links are integrated into the concept map.

7. Refinement process integrates changes in the concept map structure.

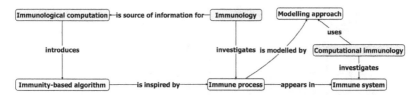

Fig. 18: Backbone of the concept map ComImmuno-AIS (adjusted from (Husáková, 2015c))

The following Fig. 19 depicts the concept map in the first version where concepts and cross-links of immunology, artificial immune systems and computational immunology are represented. All of these application domains are highly complex. This is the reason why the most important concepts and relations are integrated.

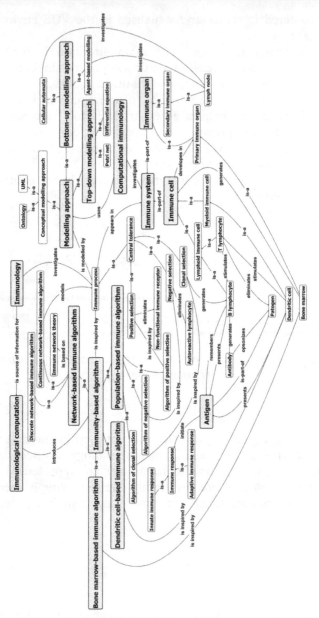

Fig. 19: The first version of the concept map ComImmuno-AIS (adjusted from (Husáková, 2015c))

6.1.2 Concept map as repository for topic map development

Concept maps are visualised with various software tools. These tools often offer a support for browsing their content with querying. The Topic Maps is the international standard ISO/IEC 13250 Topic Maps (ISO, 2008). The standard is intended to realise the ideas of the semantic web - to offer intelligent tools for improvement navigation and searching relevant information/knowledge as fast as possible without the information overload of the final user. The Topic Maps standard defines knowledge representation schema composed of three main elements - topic, association and occurrence. Topic is computer representation of some object of our interest. Association represents relations between these topics and occurrence represents information sources explaining the topic in more detail. Information sources can be internal (typically definition or description) or external (typically web source). Each of these elements has a specific class – a type. Having these elements, the Topic Maps document represents the metadata layer above the existing digital sources of different types.

The ComImmuno-AIS concept map is used as a basis for topic map representation. Development of the topic map is divided on representation of the ontology - hierarchical structure containing topic types, association types and occurrence types. The types are identified with the usage of the ComImmuno-AIS concept map. The Linear Topic Map Notation (LTM) syntax is used for the topic map development (Garshol, 2006). It is the non-standardised syntax that can represent content of the topic map in short piece of code. Fig. 20 presents the piece of the code written in the LTM syntax. The topic map-based ontology is depicted in Fig. 21 where the core topic types are in grey rectangles.

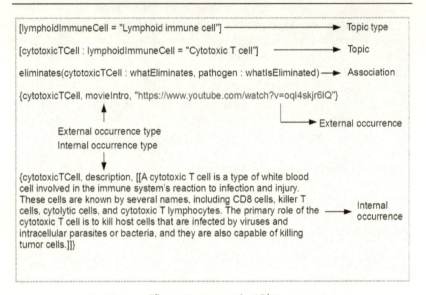

Fig. 20: The topic map - the LTM syntax

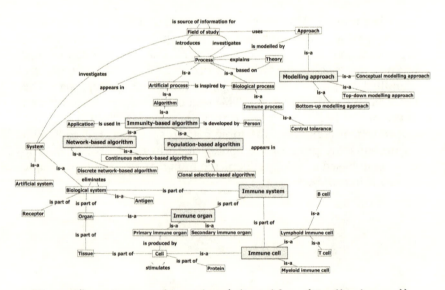

Fig. 21: The topic map - the ontology (adjusted from (Husáková, 2015c))

The Ontopia open-source environment is used for management of the developed topic map (Ontopia [n. d.]). Omnigator is used for verification of the LTM-based topic map and browsing its content. Vizigator is applied for visualising the structure of the topic map and query plugin is used for querying the content of the topic map where the query language Tolog is used. Fig. 22 depicts the three-based view on the topic map with the usage of the Omnigator browser.

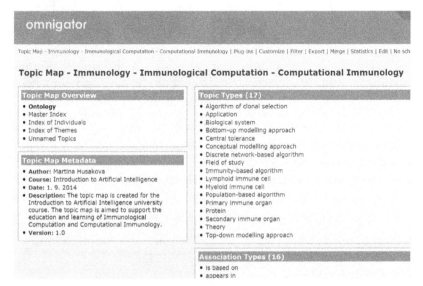

Fig. 22: The ComImmuno-AIS in the Omnigator

The actual LTM-based topic map contains 17 topic types, 16 association types, 10 external occurrence types, 8 internal occurrence types, 152 topics, 83 associations between topics, 129 external occurrences and 32 internal occurrences.

6.2   ENTITY-RELATIONSHIP DIAGRAMS

Entity-relationship modelling is used for abstract and conceptual representation of data. This method of data modelling specifies conceptual schema of the information system mainly based on a relational database. Entity-relationship diagram (ERD) is a graphical representation of the entity-relationship model and it is designed in the early stages of the database development. The database is represented as a collection of entity types, relations between them and attributes with their values. Entity type is a collection of entities sharing the same or similar characteristics. Example of the entity type can be: a protein, a gene, a receptor, a chemokine, etc. Entity is the concrete example (the instance) of the entity type. Example of the entity can be: HER2 (a gene), MHC-II (a receptor), IL-1 (a cytokine), etc. Attributes with values are data we wish to store about entity types, i. e. entities. Example of the attribute can be: identification value of the acid, name of the surface molecule, shape of the cell, etc. One or more attributes can be used as primary keys for entities identification. Entity-relationship model is used for relational model development where entity types are represented by tables, entities are row of tables and attributes are columns of tables. Fig. 23 depicts the example of the ERD used for biological application domain. Non-traditional usage of the ERDs is mentioned in (Bornberg-Bauer and Paton, 2002) where relations between enzymes, their reactions with protein properties and biopolymers are modelled.

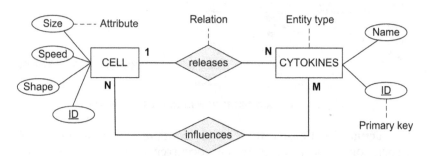

Fig. 23: Example of the ERD - Cells and cytokines

6.3   ONTOLOGIES

Ontology has the origin in philosophy (metaphysics). It is focused on human being in the philosophical point of view. It tries to answer on questions related to the living or non-living things existing in our world, e. g. what the existence is, what is the purpose of the things which are around us, what relations exist between these things, etc. Ontologies are perceived as knowledge-based structures in the context of the computer science - ontological engineering. Ontological engineering is the subarea of the knowledge engineering that is interested in all activities related to development of knowledge-based applications (knowledge retrieval, knowledge representation, knowledge sharing, knowledge maintenance). American computer scientist J. McCarthy presented ontologies in relation with the common-sense knowledge - routine (often inaccurate) pieces of knowledge which are received during our everyday lives (McCarthy, 1987). It is expected that the person has this type of knowledge and uses it in solving of typical problems. This kind of knowledge is often very general and should be integrated into the knowledge-based application. This application should not fail due to the incapability in solving "trivial" problems. Various definitions of ontologies as knowledge-based structures exist. T. Gruber specified one of the most famous explanations what the ontology is in 1993: *"Ontology is explicit specification of the conceptualisation."* (Gruber, 1993). Ontologies should be represented explicitly, i. e. they should not be hidden in human mind. Conceptualisation corresponds with the identification of the most important concepts which should be integrated into our ontology in respect to the purpose of our model. W. Borst extended the definition of T. Gruber in (Borst, 1997): *"Ontology is formal, explicit specification of shared conceptualisation."* This definition is closer to the fulfilment of the ideas which are behind the semantic web (Lacy, 2005) initiative because of the formality and shareability of ontologies. Formal ontologies are necessary for their usage as machine-interpretable structures. Intelligent agents moving and browsing the web space need "to understand the information" located in the web documents for receiving relevant information for the final user as fast as possible. Intelligent agents often need to communicate with each other during problem solving in the web space. Communication is often based on the information/knowledge of the agent. Ontologies play the role of the vocabulary of "things" with the meaning which is used by the agent as a knowledge base for problem solving and communication with other intelligent agents. Intelligent agents require formal representation of these vocabularies. Formal ontologies are often expressed in RDF (Resource Description Framework), RDF(S) or

OWL (Ontology Web Language) - formal languages used in metadata representation for web documents (RDF, RDF(S)) and for knowledge representation in web ontologies (OWL). Shareability of ontologies corresponds with the possibility to present pieces of knowledge in public space, e. g. for community of interested persons who require compact knowledge repository for problem solving and decision making. The ontology is more or less complex structure used for (Uschold and Gruninger, 1996):

- information or knowledge sharing between people,
- information or knowledge sharing between machines (intelligent agents),
- information or knowledge sharing between people and machines,
- reusing general or domain-specific pieces of knowledge,
- analysis of the application domain and for software development,
- development of knowledge bases for knowledge-based systems,
- representation of vocabulary for communication between machines.

In the view of the computational immunology, bio-ontologies are specific classes of ontologies representing (bio)medical pieces of knowledge. They play the central role in information and knowledge integration about various organisms. These ontologies are then saved into databases and accessed to support their sharing and communication between interested parties. The bio-ontologies are defined in (Robinson and Bauer, 2011) as: "... *tools for annotation and data integration that provide bench researchers with a common vocabulary to describe and communicate results and give bioinformaticians tools for the functional analysis of microarray data, network modeling, semantic similarity for biological analysis and clinical diagnostics, as well as many other applications.*" OBO Foundry (Open Biological and Biomedical Ontologies) is the collaborative experiment with the goal to develop biomedicine-based ontologies and provide the space where it is possible to find and share bio-ontologies. The initiative is under patronage of NCBO (National Center for Biomedical Ontology) and offers the repository of bio-ontologies. Minority of them are "OBO Foundry ontologies" which have been already accepted by OBO foundry community. Majority of them are OBO Foundry candidates or other ontologies of interest. Gene ontology (GO) is one of the best known OBO foundry ontologies. It became the standard in bio-medical ontologies. It is a part of the Gene Ontology project - bioinformatics initiative having the goal to standardise genes representation and gene products of various organisms. GO offers controlled vocabulary of terms for annotation gene products without distinguishing animal species. Cellular components, molecular functions and biological processes are main domains which are covered by GO (Ashburner et al., 2000). The GO can be visualised with the OLSVis software, see Fig. 24 visualising the term the immune system. BioPortal offers the repository of ontologies from the biological and medical domains (Whetzel et al., 2011). It enables to browse the content of ontologies and visualises their structure. The cell ontology is one of the example of ontologies that are accessed in the BioPortal. The cell ontology is focused on representation of various cell types independent on the organism. It represents knowledge about prokaryotic organisms and eukaryotic organisms in the directed acyclic graph. Figure 25 depicts various terms and related information in the graph structure.

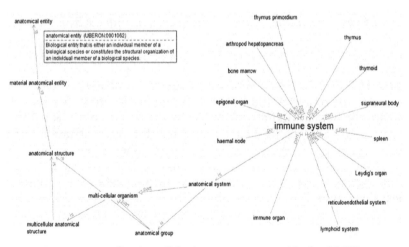

Fig. 24: Visualisation of the immune system with the OLSVis

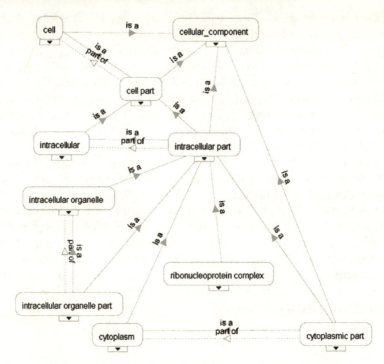

Fig. 25: Visualisation of the intracellular parts with the BioPortal

The HBVO (Human Biological Viruses Ontology) ontology is focused on representation of various types of viruses which can attack the human (Raffat, 2012). The aim of this ontology is to offer structured and controlled vocabulary for categorisation and description of biological viruses. Virus taxonomy defined by the International Committee on Taxonomy of Viruses was used for ontology development. Fig. 26 (adopted from (Raffat, 2012), Fig. 4) visualises graphical structure of the HBVO ontology (Raffat, 2012).

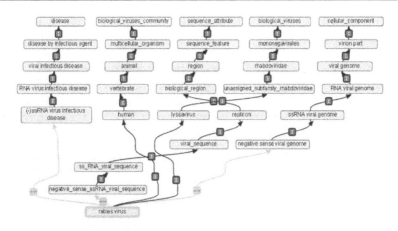

Fig. 26: Structure of the HBVO ontology (adopted from (Raffat, 2012), Fig. 4)

The AIS-OWL ontology was developed with the aim to offer the view on the artificial immune systems and related research areas (Husáková, 2010). The content of the ontology is focused on the approaches of AIS modelling, immunity-based algorithms with their usage, immune cells and immune processes. The universal framework modelling structure of the artificial immune systems plays the role of a guidance for the AIS-OWL ontology development, see Fig. 27 (adopted from (de Castro and Timmis, 2002), Fig. 3.1).

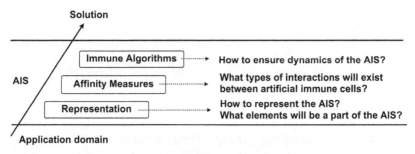

Fig. 27: Layered framework of the AIS (adopted from (de Castro and Timmis, 2002), Fig. 3.1)

The AIS-OWL ontology is developed in the Protégé-OWL tool (ver. 3.3.1) in normalised shape. It contains 155 primitive classes, 22 definable classes, 251 existential, 46 universal restrictions and 24 object properties. This ontology is related to the work of colleagues from Wuhan University in China (Tao et al., 2008). They used DAML language for developing of the ontology about the artificial immune systems. This ontology integrates several models and algorithms of the artificial immune systems. Fig. 28 depicts the fragment of the AIS-OWL ontology visualising the taxonomy of artificial processes and biological processes.

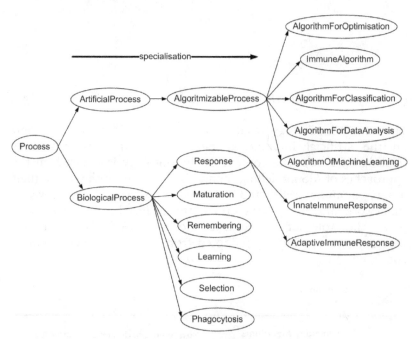

Fig. 28: Fragment of the AIS-OWL ontology - Processes

6.4   SBML

Systems Biology Markup Language is a machine-readable format for representing models (Hucka et al., 2003). The language is based on the extensible markup language (XML) and mainly used for modelling cell signalling pathways, metabolic pathways, biochemical reactions or gene regulatory networks. The main motivation behind the SBML is to offer declarative language for modelling biological systems and processes occurring inside them. There existed various notations for depicting biological phenomena in the past, but they were in contradiction to each other. The SBML is one of the attempts for avoiding this problem. The SBML does not play the role of the universal language for models representation. It is a format independent on software tools that is used for reading or writing biology-based models. The SBML is completely free and open for updating and proposing the extensions. It is de facto standard in the systems biology. The language has three levels coexisting with each other (Finney and Hucka, 2003):

- SBML Level 1: This version was proposed in 2001. It offers elementary possibilities for modelling biological compartments (2001).
- SBML Level 2: This version was proposed in 2003. It offers some extensions for specification of the SBML-based models:
  o MathML language is used for expression of the mathematical formulas.
  o User defined functions, events and constraints are supported.
  o Compartments types and species types are supported.
  o Structure of rules is simplified.
- SBML Level 3: This version was introduced in the final release specification in 2010 and specifies the following and others proposals:
  o Data structures for non-deterministic modelling (e. g. Petri nets, markov chains, probability models) are supported.
  o Arrays and sets are supported.
  o Controlled vocabulary can be used for synonyms representation.

The most general interpretation of the SBML-based models is based on the idea where the investigated system is represented as a set of compartments where biological entities "lives". These entities are

linked by processes transforming one entity into another entity or
influencing a position of the entity, see Fig. 29.

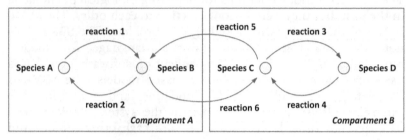

Fig. 29: General interpretation of the SBML-based model

Structure of the SBML-based models is different with respect to the
level of the SBML. Structure of the SBML model (Level 2) is divided
on several sections – lists. All lists are optional and their order is
significant (Hucka et al., 2003):

- Beginning of the XML file – declaration of the XML
  document
    - Beginning of the SBML model definition
        - List of function definitions (new in the Level 2)
        - List of unit definitions
        - List of compartments types (new in the Level 2)
        - List of species types (new in the Level 2)
        - List of compartments
        - List of species
        - List of parameters
        - List of initial assignments (new in the Level 2)
        - List of rules
        - List of constraints (new in the Level 2)
        - List of reactions
        - List of events (new in the Level 2)
    - End of the SBML model definition

<Function definitions> section contains named mathematical
functions that are represented by MathML lambda objects. These
functions can be used on the various places of the SBML model.
<Unit definitions> section contains declaration of the new used unit
of measurement or redefinition of the default unit of measurement.

<Compartment> represents a container for biological entities called species. It specifies a place where the biological entity is located (e. g. a cell, a nucleus, a mitochondria). Species are biological/chemical entities contained in the compartments (e. g. nucleic acids, proteins, genes, ions). Each species have to be a part of some compartment. <Classes of compartments and species> are called types. They collect compartments and species sharing the similar or the same characteristics. <List of parameters> contains parameters of the biological system. The following parameters are distinguished in the SBML: constants, variables, local parameters and global parameters (Hucka et al., 2003). Initial conditions of the SBML model are mentioned in the section <list of initial assignments>. <List of rules> contains restrictions on the SBML model (variables, parameters) for cases in which constraints cannot be expressed with the usage of the reaction components. <Reaction section> defines actions related to the biological entities and occurred in the biological system, e. g. transformation processes, transportation processes or binding processes. Changes in the amount of species are one of the outputs of reactions. <List of reactions> contains list of reactants and products as the outputs of the reactions. <List of events> describes changes in a set of variables of any type (e. g. changes in the quantity of the species, a size of a compartment or parameters of the SBML model).

The SBML language is not intended to read by humans or written by hand. It should be used by computer as machine-readable format for exchanging information about investigated biological system. The following simple example (Example 1) demonstrates the notation of the SBML document. The SBML document starts with the core element – tag <xml> and specification of the xml version and encoding. The following rooted tag <sbml> introduces the name space for the particular version of the SBML. "Starting point" of the SBML model is represented by the tag <model> with an identification value and a name. This paired tag defines a container for all lists mentioned above.

Example 1: Backbone of the SBML document

```
<?xml version="1.0" encoding="UTF-8"?>
<sbml xmlns="http://www.sbml.org/sbml/level2/version4" level="2" version="4">
<model id="DemoExample" name="Example of the SBML document">
    ...
    ...
</model>
</sbml>
```

The following example (Example 2) extends the backbone of the SBML document mentioned in the Example 1 with the particular lists. The compartments should be defined by a paired tag <listOfCompartments>. The list contains specific compartments for species. The Example 2 represents couple of compartments of the cell: a cell, a membrane, a cytoplasm, a nucleus and a mitochondria. Each of them can have some additional attributes, but the id attribute is mandatory. Relations between compartments is defined by the <outside> attribute. It models topological associations between parts of the whole.

Example 2: The SBML document - compartments

```
<listOfCompartments>
    <compartment id="bloodStream" name="Blood stream"/>
    <compartment id="cell" name="Cell" size="1" outside="bloodStream"/>
    <compartment id="cytoplasm" name="Cytoplasm" outside="cell"/>
    <compartment id="nucleus" name="Nucleus" outside="cytoplasm"/>
    <compartment id="mitochondria" name="Mitochondria" outside="cytoplasm"/>
</listOfCompartments>
```

List of species is represented with the paired tag <listOfSpecies>. The declaration of species is similar to the compartments representation, see Example 3. Each species has an identification value (id) and a name as attribute. Compartment attribute indicates a location for the species. Initial amount attribute represents amount of species in the beginning of the simulation.

Example 3: The SBML document - species

```
<listOfSpecies>
    <species id="mRNA" name="mRNA" compartment="nucleus"
    initialAmount="0.00328"/>
    <species id="RNA" name="RNA" compartment="cytoplasm"
    initialAmount="0.0054"/>
    <species id="ab" name="Antibody" compartment="bloodStream"/>
    <species id="ag" name="Antigen" compartment="bloodStream"/>
    <species id="ab-agComplex" name="Antibody-Antigen complex"
    compartment="bloodStream"/>
</listOfSpecies>
```

The following Example 4 extends the previous one. It adds the next container representing possible reactions between species. Formation of antibody-antigen complex is selected as an example. List of reactions is represented with the paired tag <listOfReactions>. Particular reaction is represented by the paired tag <reaction> with an id and a name attribute. List of reactants (paired tag <listOfReactants>) (biological entities – species interacting with each other) and list of products (paired tag <listOfProducts>) (outputs of interactions between species) is the nested structure of the paired tag <reaction>.

Example 4: The SBML document - reactions

```
<listOfReactions>
    <reaction id="Ab-AgBinding" name="Antibody-Antigen complex formation">
    <listOfReactants>
        <speciesReference species="ab"/>
        <speciesReference species="ag"/>
    </listOfReactants>
    <listOfProducts>
        <speciesReference species="ab-agComplex"/>
    </listOfProducts>
    </reaction>
</listOfReactions>
```

SBML documents can be visualised with the aid of various tools. The CellDesigner is structured diagram editor used mainly (but not limited) for drawing biochemical networks (Funahashi et al., 2007). Networks are represented by the process diagrams using the graphical notation proposed by H. Kitano (Kitano, 2003), see the list of proposed elements in the appendix A (Kitano et al. [n. d.]), (Kitano, 2003).

Process diagram is a state-transition diagram consisting of the nodes and arcs. Nodes represent states of molecules or complexes. Arcs represent changes in states of molecules. The CellDesigner supports the SBML notation and offer a possibility to create and edit SBML-based files with the usage of GUI. Fig. 30 is the graphical representation of the SBML document that was mentioned above. The CellDesigner visualises compartments of the cell (cytoplasm, mitochondria, nucleus) with two nucleic acids (mRNA, RNA) and a reaction between antibody and antigen in Fig. 30. The CellDesigner is not intended only for graphical representation of biological systems and processes, but it also integrates SBML ODE Solver and Copasi tool for simulations.

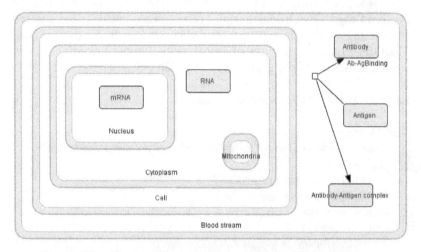

Fig. 30: Visualisation of the SBML document in the CellDesigner

Cytoscape is the next very known software platform used for visualisation biological systems (Shannon et al., 2003). Originally, the Cytoscape was intended for biological research, but it became the general tool used for analysis and visualisation of complex networks. The first version was made public in 2003. The Cytoscape 3 offers the new GUI and advanced functions. Cytoscape.js is a free and open-source javascript library also used for visualisation and analysis of complex networks. It can be used for networks integration into the own applications. Its functionality can be extended by plugins. The CySBML is the plugin for the Cytoscape 2.8 developed by M. König and A. Dräger (Center for Bioinformatics Tuebingen) (Konig et al., 2012). It supports various formats, e. g. OBO (The Open Biological and Biomedical Ontologies), GraphML (The Graph File Format), BioPAX (Biological Pathways Exchange) or SBML. It offers the import of the SBML files and visualisation and analysis of their structure. Various layouts help with receiving different views on the investigated network structure. Interface of the CySBML is very simple. It offers the options for import of the SBML files, import of files from the BioModels database and validation of SBML documents. Fig. 31 depicts the visualisation of the regulatory system of the T-cell in the Cytoscape 2.8.0 (CySBML), (Alexander and Wahl, 2011). It depicts the state transitions between proteins (circles, diamonds (degraded proteins)) involved into the regulatory processes. Various reactions between proteins are included, e. g. suppression, death, maturation or activation.

Biographer is a visualisation tool for analysis of biological networks developed at the Theoretical Biophysics Group in Berlin (Krause et al., 2013). It uses layout algorithms optimizing layout of graphs of biological networks in a web browser. It can be used as an editor of the SBML files where the structure of the biological network can be created by hand. It offers a possibility to import SBML files and visualises their structure. Export of SBML files into graphical formats is also possible. Fig. 32 (Alexander and Wahl, 2011) depicts the visualisation of the regulation system of the T-cell in the Biographer.

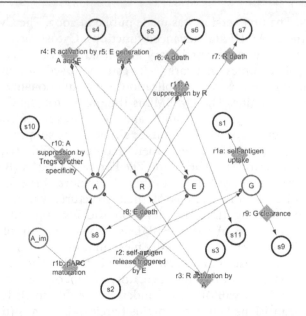

Fig. 31: Regulation system of the T-cell in the CySBML plugin (Alexander and Wahl, 2011)

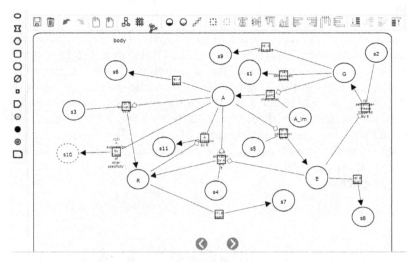

Fig. 32: Regulation system of the T-cell in the Biographer (Alexander and Wahl, 2011)

Biographer is used as visualisation tool in the semanticSBML software written in Python language (Krause et al., 2010), see Fig. 33. It offers collection of tools used for analysis of biological networks. It is possible to search the BioModels.net database, cluster models by their annotation similarities and visualised them as graph structures, compare of different versions of the SBML models from the BioModels.net database or annotate of SBML models.

View SBML model
Display SBML models visually

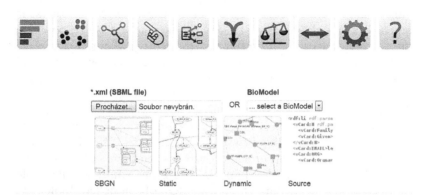

Fig. 33: semanticSBML - main screen (semanticSBML 2.0)

6.5 SBGN

SBGN (Systems Biology Graphical Notation) is a graphical notation developed by a wide community of biochemists, modellers and computer scientists. The SBGN project was initiated in 2005 with the aim to develop and standardise systematic and unambiguous notation for transformation of biological pieces of knowledge into the more formal shape (Le Novere et al., 2009). Previous notations used in biology or medicine were developed in "ad hoc style". Ambiguous of used elements of various notations was the result of this approach. The SBGN notation is composed of three languages. Each of the language focuses on different aspect of the biological system. The following three languages are distinguished in the SBGN notation:

- The Process description language (PD), (level 1, version 1.0 (2008)), (see appendix B) (Le Novère et al., 2008),
- Entity relationship language (ER) (level 1, version 1.0 (2009)), (see appendix C), (Le Novère et al., 2009),
- Activity flow language (AF) (level 1, version 1.0 (2009)), (see appendix D) (Mi et al., 2009).

6.5.1 Process description language

The Process description language is focused on modelling molecular processes changing states of the biological entities. It represents how the biological entity changes its state in response to the particular process. It means that the biological entity can occur several times in the diagram. Changes in states relate with temporal aspects of processes. The Process description diagram (the map) is able to integrate temporal characteristics of processes. The Process description diagram is useful e. g. for modelling of temporal pathways of biochemical interactions occurring in biochemical networks or for modelling of metabolic pathways. The PD takes the inspiration from the processes-based notations used in the CellDesigner and from the Edinburgh Pathway Notation (EPN) able to deal with an incomplete knowledge of modelled biological pathways (Moodie et al., 2006). The PD defines six classes of glyphs in the level 1 (Le Novere et al., 2009):

1. Entity pool nodes, auxiliary units: an unspecified entity, a simple chemical entity, a macromolecule, a feature of a nucleid acid, a perturbing agent, multimers, a source sink, a complex, a unit of information, a state variable.
2. Process nodes: a process itself, an omitted process, an uncertain process, an association, a dissociation, a phenotype.
3. Container nodes: a compartment.
4. Reference nodes: a submap, a tag.
5. Connecting arcs: a consumption, a production, a modulation, a stimulation, a catalysis, an inhibition, a necessary stimulation, a logic arc, an equivalence arc.
6. Logical operators: and operator, or operator and not operator.

Complex formation is a typical problem that can be represented with the usage of the PD. Fig. 34 (adjusted from (SBGNDictionary [n. d.])) depicts the general view on the basic SBGN elements that can be used for modelling complex formation. There are two macromolecules (X, Y) forming the complex consisting of these two macromolecules. The macromolecule SBGN-PD element is used for macromolecules representation. Macromolecule is a very large molecule with high relative molecular mass composed of smaller units. It is built up from covalent linking of pseudo-identical units (Le Novère et al., 2008). Complex formation is modelled with the association SBGN-PD element - a connecting arc used for representation of non-covalent binding of the biological entities forming larger complex (Le Novère et al., 2008). The process node association is related with the two next connecting arcs. The first one is the consumption ingoing arc. This SBGN-PD element represents the fact that the entity pool (X, Y) is consumed ("used") by a particular process (formation). The second one is the production outgoing arc. This SBGN-PD element represents the fact that the entity pool (X, Y) is produced by a particular process (formation). The complex SBGN element represents complex consisting of two macromolecules (X, Y). Complex is a complex node representing biochemical entity consisting of other biochemical entities. It is represented by specific container including smaller biochemical entities.

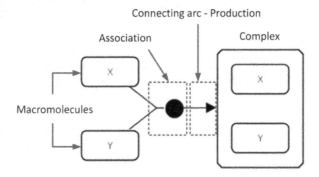

Fig. 34: Complex formation (PD) - general view (adjusted from (SBGNDictionary [n. d.]))

Formation of haemoglobin is the concrete example relating with the complex formation, see Fig. 35 (adjusted from (Le Novère et al., 2009), Fig. 2.28). The PD map contains haem. Haem is represented as a simple chemical. Simple chemical SBGN-PD element is represented as circular container. It is a chemical compound that is not formed by the covalent linking of pseudo-identical residues (Le Novère et al., 2008). The haem has the association with the globin macromolecule SBGN-PD element. Combination of haem and globin forms the complex haemoglobin with the consumption and production connecting arcs. The complex heamoblogin is visualised with the complex SBGN-PD element. Formation of complete haemoglobin is represented with the combination of consumption and production connecting arcs. Combination of the haem and the globin complete haemoglobin.

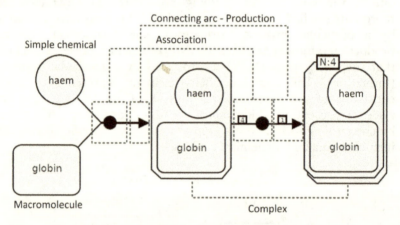

Fig. 35: Complex formation (PD) - formation of haemoglobin (adjusted from (Le Novère et al., 2009), Fig. 2.28)

6.5.2 Entity relationships language

The Entity relationships language is not focused on the states of entities and their transformations caused by the various biological (biochemical) processes. The ER models biological entities and how they affect each other. It tries to answer the question how the biological entities influence each other and how this influence has the effects on biological entities (Le Novère et al., 2009). Relations between entities are viewed as rules representing influences of biological entities on different relations. The biological entity is the main concept of the ER in comparison to the PD, where the process is in the centre of the interest. Entity is occurred only once in this diagram (a map). The temporal characteristics cannot be easily represented by the Entity relationships diagram (map) or sequences of "biological events" in comparison to the Process description language (Le Novere et al., 2009). The ER is suitable for modelling of signalling pathways. The ER takes the inspiration from the Molecular Interaction Maps (MIM) notation used for representation of biological networks containing various proteins, multi-protein complexes or enzymes (Kohn, 1999). The ER defines five classes of glyphs in the level 1 (Le Novère et al., 2009):

1. Entity nodes, auxiliary units: an entity, outcome of an entity, a perturbing agent, a unit of information, a state variable, an existence, a location.
2. Logical operators: and operator, or operator, not operator and delay operator.
3. Reference nodes: annotation.
4. Statements: an assignment, an interaction, a non-interaction, an observable.
5. Influences: a modulation, a stimulation, a necessary stimulation, an absolute stimulation, an inhibition, an absolute inhibition, a logic arc.

Complex formation can be represented also with the usage of the ER of the SBGN. The general view on the complex formation is depicted on Fig. 36. Entity nodes (X, Y) represent biological entities. The ER distinguishes three entity nodes: the interactors, the logical operators and the perturbing agent (Le Novère et al., 2009). The interactor is the entity node (biological entity) able to interact with the environment. The ER distinguishes two types of interactors: entities and outcomes of a statement. Three interactors are depicted on Fig. 36 (two entities (X, Y) and one outcome represented as a filled dot). Existence state variable contains the result of interaction between entities (X, Y). Assignment SBGN-ER element is a statement that is able to set the state variable to a concrete value. Existence is the example of the state variable containing a result thanks to the assignment and the stimulation SBGN-ER element. Stimulation is a type of influence that positively affects the strength or the probability of the target relationship (Le

Novère et al., 2009). The delay SBGN-ER element is a logical operator able to represent time delays in biological processes. This SBGN-ER element is used also in Fig. 36. Possible delays can exist because complex formation (X_Y) can take some time. The ER does not contain the complex element in comparison to the SBGN-PD, but the complex is represented as the entity node (X_Y) in Fig. 36.

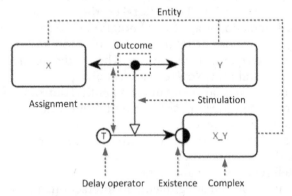

Fig. 36: Complex formation (ER) - general view (adjusted from (SBGNDictionary [n. d.]))

6.5.3 Activity flow language

The Activity flow language (AF) models information flow between biological entities in biological networks, i. e. it focuses on representation of relations between activities of biological entities. It is mainly useful for description of signalling pathways or gene regulatory networks. It defines the following five classes of glyphs in the level 1 (Mi et al., 2009):

1. Activity nodes: a biological activity, a phenotype, a perturbation.
2. Auxiliary units: a macromolecule, a simple chemical, a genetic, an unspecified, a complex.
3. Modulating arcs: positive influence, negative influence, unknown influence, necessary stimulation.
4. Logical operators: <and> operator, <or> operator, <not> operator, delay.
5. Container nodes: a compartment.

The complex formation can be represented also with the AF, see Fig. 37. The main attention is paid for the biological activities in comparison to the PD and ER. The crucial elements are two biological activities (X, Y) responsible for the resulted biological activity (complex formation, X_Y) in Fig. 37. Biological activity is the SBGN-AF activity node representing activities of biological entities. The biological activity node can contain the unit of information – the smaller box above the biological activity SBGN-AF element. This box often contains the concrete name of the biological entity which is responsible for the activity, e. g. a simple chemical or a macromolecule. This box is empty in Fig. 37. Logic arc SBGN-AF element models the fact that the activity influences the outcome of the particular logic operator, the AND logic operator in the case of complex formation in Fig. 37. The logic operator AND models the situation in which all activities of X and Y are necessary for influencing the target activity X_Y in the case of complex formation. The positive influence is the SBGN-AF modulation arc representing the positive influence on the following activity X_Y in case of the complex formation.

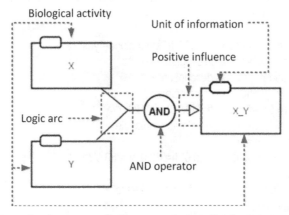

Fig. 37: Complex formation (AF) - general view (SBGNDictionary [n. d.])

The SBGN notation is supported by various software tools, e. g. CellDesigner, Cytoscape (plugin CySBGN), Athena, Arcadia or Biographer. The SBGN-ML is the XML implementation of the SBGN. The SBGN-ML is supported by several software tools, especially by VANTED (SBGN-ED), PathVisio, Systems Biology

Workbench or Render Comparison. The libSBGN is the library dealing also with the SBGN-ML file format. The Example 5 (adopted from (SBGNDictionary [n. d.])) mentions the source code written in the SBGN-ML. This piece of code is the computational representation of the complex formation. The SBGN-ML document starts with the XML declaration (<xml>) and usage of the <sbgn> tag introducing the root tag as a container for SBGN-based elements. The <map> tag with the attribute language specifies the used SBGN language ("process description" for PD, "entity relationship" for ER and "activity flow" for AF). Particular SBGN element is represented with the <glyph> tag. Each of the glyph has the attribute id and class. The id attribute represents a unique identification value for each glyph. The class attribute specifies the concrete SBGN element, e. g. complex, macromolecule, association, production, consumption, etc. The <glyph> tag represents a container including specific characteristics of the element, e. g. name, graphical representation of the element or nested biological elements, see Example 5 (adopted from (SBGNDictionary [n. d.])) .

Example 5: Complex formation in the SBGN-ML (adopted from (SBGNDictionary [n. d.]))

```
<?xml version="1.0" encoding="UTF-8" standalone="yes"?>
<sbgn xmlns="http://sbgn.org/libsbgn/0.2">
   <map language="process description">
      <glyph id="glyph0" class="complex">
   <bbox y="10.0" x="200.0" h="160.0" w="120.0"/>
         <glyph id="glyph3" class="macromolecule">
            <label text="X"/>
            <bbox y="30.0" x="220.0" h="40.0" w="80.0"/>
         </glyph>
         <glyph id="glyph2" class="macromolecule">
            <label text="Y"/>
            <bbox y="110.0" x="220.0" h="40.0" w="80.0"/>
         </glyph>
      </glyph>
      <glyph id="glyph4" class="macromolecule">
         <label text="X"/>
         <bbox y="20.0" x="10.0" h="40.0" w="80.0"/>
      </glyph>
```

```
<glyph id="glyph1" class="macromolecule">
  <label text="Y"/>
  <bbox y="120.0" x="10.0" h="40.0" w="80.0"/>
</glyph>
<glyph id="glyph5" class="association">
  <bbox y="78.0" x="128.0" h="24.0" w="24.0"/>
  <port y="90.0" x="164.0" id="glyph5.2"/>
  <port y="90.0" x="116.0" id="glyph5.1"/>
</glyph>
<arc target="glyph0" source="glyph5.2" id="arc0" class="production">
  <start y="90.0" x="164.0"/>
  <end y="90.0" x="200.0"/>
</arc>
<arc target="glyph5.1" source="glyph4" id="arc1" class="consumption">
  <start y="60.0" x="76.4"/>
  <end y="90.0" x="116.0"/>
</arc>
<arc target="glyph5.1" source="glyph1" id="arc2" class="consumption">
  <start y="120.0" x="76.4"/>
  <end y="90.0" x="116.0"/>
</arc>
  </map>
</sbgn>
```

6.6 CellML

CellML is the open standard based on the XML language. It is developed by the Auckland Bioengineering Institute at the University of Auckland. CellML is primarily used for description of cellular biological systems with the usage of mathematical expressions, i. e. ordinary differential equations, differential algebraic equations or simple linear algebra (Hedley and Nelson, 2001). The CellML can be used for modelling various scales of cellular systems. The CellML is declarative language mainly applied for development, storage and sharing mathematical models of cellular biological systems with other developers. The CellML is distributed in version 1.0 (Hedley and Nelson, 2001) and 1.1. (Cuellar et al., 2006). The possibility to import particular components and units of different CellML-based models and reuse them for specific purposes is the main difference between these two versions. The CellML uses component-based architecture that facilitates to reuse components in various CellML-based models. The CellML-based cellular models use the MathML – XML-based language for expression of cellular processes in terms of mathematics. Metadata information can enrich the CellML models for additional information that are able to help with decision if the CellML model is suitable for particular needs of the modeller. Metadata are encoded by the RDF (Resource Description Framework). The CellML cannot be used only for description of cellular systems quantitatively (with mathematical description of cellular processes), but the CellML can be useful also for representation of qualitative models of biological systems where relations between components are deeply explained (Lloyd et al., 2004). Visual tools can depict the logical or physical structure of the modelled cellular system. The CellML can be applied for modelling various processes which are not limited to the cell migration, signal transduction, gene regulation, immunological processes, processes occurring in the endocrine or neural system. The CellML model consists of the following sections for which the order is not significant (Hedley et al., 2001):

- Beginning of the XML file – declaration of the XML document
    - Beginning of the CellML model definition
        - Import section
        - Declaration of units
        - Representation of components
        - Specification of groups
        - Representation of connections
    - End of the Cell model definition

All elements of the CellML document are contained in the <model> root element. The <model> element has the mandatory attribute name for unique identification of the model, see Example 6. Import section contains parts that are imported from others CellML models. The <import> tag with attribute href contains URI of the CellML model from which the parts are being imported. One component (MyFirstComponent) and one unit (Inch) is imported in the Example 6. User-defined units are declared with the <units> tag. Declaration of the inch unit is also mentioned in the Example 6.

Example 6: Basic structure of the CellML document

```
<?xml version="1.0"?>
<!--MODEL DECLARATION-->
<model name="exampleDemo-01" xmlns=http://www.cellml.org/cellml/1.1#
xmlns:cellml=http://www.cellml.org/cellml/1.1#
xmlns:cmeta="http://www.cellml.org/metadata/1.0#">
<!--IMPORT DECLARATION-->
<import xlink:href="...">
<units name="Fahrenheit" units_ref="F" />
<component name="MyFirstComponent" component_ref="MyFirstComponent" />

<!--UNITS DECLARATION-->
<units name="Inch">
    <unit multiplier="2.54" prefix="centi" units="metre" />
</units>
...

...
</import>
</model>
```

The <component> tag represents component – a compact functional unit that is similar to the concept of a class in the UML language, see the subchapter 6.8. The component consists of block with variables and block of equations with mathematical expressions manipulating with variables. A component can be defined in the model or import section. A component is uniquely identified by its name – the name attribute is used for this purpose. Various biological entities can be represented by a component, e. g. a cellular membrane, a mitochondria, a T-cell, an antibody, a sodium channel, an environment in which the cell moves, etc. Structure of a component is similar to the UML class. It contains the following sections:

- units of component,
- variables specify properties of a component,
- reactions represent particular reactions that are part of specific cellular pathway,
- mathematical expressions (equations) modify values of variables.

Behaviour of modelled cellular system can be mathematically described with the mathematical equations. MathML is the XML-based language used for the representation of mathematical expressions. Mathematical equations are expressed in the <mathml:math> root tag. The Example 7 introduces the representation of very simple equation X = (10 * (Y + Z)) – 100 where the <ci> tag represents variable, <cn> tag represents number (a constant value) and <apply> tag is used for application of particular mathematical operators (e. g. plus, minus, times, division, factorial, etc.), trigonometric operators (e. g. sin, cos, tan, etc.), logic operators (e. g. and, or, not, xor) and many others.

Example 7: Equation in the CellML document

```
<mathml:math id="001" xmlns="http://www.w3.org/1998/Math/MathML">
    <apply id="Mathematical_example_001"><eq />
    <ci>X</ci>
        <apply><times/>
            <cn cellml:units="celsius">10</cn>
            <apply><plus/>
                <ci>Y</ci>
                <ci>Z</ci>
            </apply>
        </apply><minus/>
        <cl>100</cl>
    </apply>
```

Section with connections is the next segment that is a part of the CellML document. Connections offer the possibility to exchange pieces of information between components. It can be viewed as a mechanism for communication between components. A connection contains all variables that are going to be mapped between components. Interface concept plays very important role for connections realisation. Transferred variable value from the first component has to be declared with the interface containing the attribute value out. Interface declaration is a part of a component. The second component that "wants" to receive the variable value contains a declaration of this variable together with the interface with the attribute value in. Two components (the membrane and the sodium channel) are represented in the Example 8 (adopted from (Cuellar et al., 2006)). These components dispose variable V that is available for transferring from the membrane component (public_interface="out"). The sodium_channel component is able to receive value of a variable V (public_interface="in"). Example 9 (adopted from (Cuellar et al., 2006)) describes connections between the membrane and the sodium_channel component together with the mapped variable V. Variable values can be "transported" and used by different components, but these ones have not modify these values.

Example 8: Components of the CellML document (adopted from (Cuellar et al., 2006))

```
<component name="membrane">
    <variable name="V" public_interface="out" initial_value="-75.0"
    units="milivolt" />
</component>

<component name="sodium_channel">
    <variable name="V" public_interface="in" units="milivolt" />
</component>
```

Example 9: Connections of the CellML document (adopted from (Cuellar et al., 2006))

```
<connection>
    <map_components component_1="membrane"
    component_2="sodium_channel" />
    <map_variables variable_1="V" variable_2="V" />
</connection>
```

CellML can represent hierarchical organisation of cellular systems (Hedley et al., 2001). Two types of hierarchical organisations are defined by the CellML: encapsulation and containment. Encapsulation relationship defines logical organisation of components inside the cellular system. Encapsulation can simplify structure of the CellML model. Containment relationship defines physical hierarchy of components in the CellML model. Example 10 introduces the simple and general usage of the encapsulation relation. The <group> tag is a container for representation of encapsulation relation between components. A relationship variable of the <relationship_ref> tag specifies type of hierarchical relationship. A <component_ref> tag with component variable value concretizes which components participate in the relationship. In the Example 10, the component X is logically related with the component A, B and C.

Example 10: Encapsulation in the CellML document

```
<group>
    <relationship_ref relationship="encapsulation" />
    <component_ref component="component_X">
    <component_ref component="component_A" />
    <component_ref component="component_B" />
    <component_ref component="component_C" />
    </component_ref>
</group>
```

The same <group> core tag is used in case of containment relationship representation. The variable value containment is used for relationship variable of the <relationship_ref> tag instead of the encapsulation, see the Example 11 where the nucleus and the mitochondria are physically related to the cell component.

Example 11: Containment in the CellML document

```
<group>
    <relationship_ref name="cell_structure" relationship="containment" />
    <component_ref component="cell">
    <component_ref component="nucleus" />
    <component_ref component=" mitochondria " />
    </component_ref>
</group>
```

The CellML is not primarily used for conceptual modelling of biological systems, but the content of the CellML document can be visualised with the usage of various tools, e. g. VirtualCell, JSim or OpenCell. The CellML can help with the understanding of hierarchical structure of components which are inside the cellular system and this understanding can be shared with various researchers for comparison. Fig. 38 (Moraru et al., 2008) depicts the visualisation of the reactions between particular proteins and others species of the complement system. The VirtualCell in ver. 5.2 is used for visualisation in this case. The main aim of this CellML model is to quantitatively understand the modulatory mechanisms of the complement system participating in the initiation of the immune response (Liu et al., 2011).

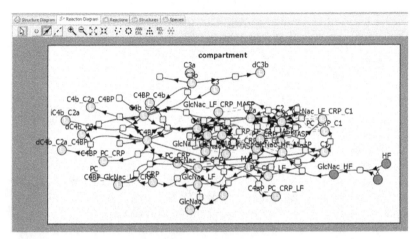

Fig. 38: Complement system in the VirtualCell (Moraru et al., 2008)

6.7 STATECHARTS

Statecharts are the extension of the state-transition diagrams (state diagrams). They are focused on graphical representation of the reactive object life-cycle or finite state machine. Finite state machine is a simple computational model representing transitions between finite number of states of the investigated system. The system changes states on the basis of symbols that are read by the system in the input. Statecharts add hierarchies of states, parallelism and communication to state-transition diagrams. Statecharts are oriented graphs where nodes represent states. A state can be perceived as time between two events. A state can have a structure consisting of an action initiated after state initialization (entry action). If the state is finished the exit action is initiated. Action Do runs during the activity of the state. Lines with arrows represent transitions between states. They model changes in states caused by the events (condition fulfilment, pressing the button, methods calling, etc.). Action does not have duration. They can be a part of transitions or inside states (entry action, do action or exit action). Fig. 39 depicts the usage of the simplified UML-based state machine diagram for modelling states of the naive T-cell when this cell enters into the paracortex of the lymph node (Abbas et al., 2011). It is supposed that the naive T-cell is alive. The mature naive state is the initial state of the naive T-cell. The mature naive T-cell attaches to the reticular fibre offering pathways for movement of the cell. If the mature naive T-cell is already attached to the reticular fibre, the cell starts to move randomly with respect to the reticular network consisting of the reticular fibres. If the mature naive T-cell is in touch with the dendritic cell it tries to recognises their surface structures – antigens on the MHC class molecule. If the recognition is successful the mature naive T-cell is stimulated and it also stimulates the dendritic cell for its activation. The mature naive T-cell becomes the mature effector T-cell and moves directly into the medullary part of the lymph node towards the efferent lymph. If the recognition of antigens on the MHC class molecule is not successful the mature naive T-cell moves randomly (Murphy et al., 2008), (Abbas et al., 2011). This is the simplification in comparison to the reality.

State-transition diagrams work on the presumption that all states of the system are known. This assumption can be true for less complex systems. State-transition diagrams are not the best choice for modelling complex systems. Statecharts proposed by D. Harel should solve the problem with complexity and should be used better for modelling complex phenomena in comparison to the state diagrams. Statecharts can be defined in the following way by D. Harel (Harel, 1987): „*Statecharts constitute a visual formalism for describing states and transitions in a modular fashion, enabling clustering, orthogonality (i. e. concurrency) and refinement, and encouraging „zoom" capabilities for moving easily back and forth between levels of abstraction.*"

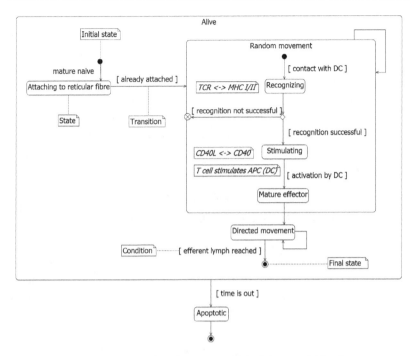

Fig. 39: Simplified domain model of the naive T-cell

Statecharts are used in conceptual modelling of the lymph node behaviour in (Swerdlin et al., 2008). These diagrams are mainly focused on representation of immune cells – B-cells, T-cells and follicular dendritic cells. Behaviour of each immune cell is depicted by the statecharts. This diagram represents inner processes of the cell and interactions with the environment. The following processes are included in the model of the lymph node: movement of cells, proliferation of cells, differentiation of B-cells into the plasmatic and memory form together with the antibodies secretion. IBM Rhapsody was used for statecharts modelling. Statecharts are also used for modelling processes occurring in the lymph node in different research study (Belkacem and Foundil, 2012). Commercial tool Anylogic was used for lymph node representation. The main attention is paid to modelling behaviour of the lymph node during the humoral immune response caused by the presence of antigens.

Spectrum of included immune cells is wider in comparison to the work of (Swerdlin et al., 2008). The following cells are taken into account in modelling behaviour of the lymph node: T_h-cells, antibodies, antigens and B-cells. The following immune processes are represented in the model:

- migration of immune cells between lymph nodes,
- immune cells cloning,
- immune cells differentiation (plasmatic cells or memory cells),
- antibodies generation.

The model is used for statistical analysis of the occupancy of the immune cells in different lymph node segments.

Biochart is the conceptual language extending the state diagrams for modelling biological systems. The language is proposed in (Kugler et al., 2010) where it is used for modelling chemotactic movement of the bacteria Escherichia Coli. IBM Rhapsody tool was applied for modelling behaviour of the bacteria.

6.8   UML

The UML (Unified Modelling Language) is standardised language mainly used during analysis and design of software applications with the usage of object-oriented approach. The UML stems from the effort to collect (merge) the best techniques used in software engineering. The UML plays the role of the unified language that is focused on the graphical representation of the object-oriented analysis and design. The UML can be defined as: *"... a graphical language for visualizing, specifying, constructing, and documenting the artifacts of a software-intensive system. The UML offers a standard way to write a system's blueprints, including conceptual things such as business processes and system functions as well as concrete things such as programming language statements, database schemas, and reusable software components."* (UML tutorial [n. d.]).

There existed several approaches for visual modelling of software systems in 1994. Method of G. Booch and J. Rumbaugh (OMT -

Object Modelling Technique) was the leading method for visual modelling of software (Arlow and Neustadt, 2005). G. Booch and J. Rumbaugh joined to the Rational Software company. They proposed the Unified Method – basis of the UML. The first version of the UML (UML 0.8) was introduced in 1995 at the OOPSLA conference. The Rational Software company bought the Objectory methodology in 1995. The UML was proposed as a standard for visual modelling with the object-oriented approach in 1996. The UML 1.1 was accepted as the industry standard for object-oriented design of software in 1997. Activites related with the improvement of the UML are under patronage of the OMG (Object Management Group) – non-profit consortium defining the UML specification. The UML was accepted as the ISO standard in 2000 and published in 2005. This version offers the accuracy improvement of the visual syntax and meta-model of the UML 1.0. The UML 2.4 was published in 2011. The UML 2.0 is divided into the four basic parts (Pilone and Pitman, 2005):

- The UML 2.0 SuperStructure: Superstructure describes the UML language in the view of the user (analytics, programmer). It describes particular diagrams with their elements.
- The UML 2.0 Infrastructure: The meta-model defines the basic elements of the language and its architecture. It specifies the core of the UML. The core of the UML uses specific packages with profiles used for the customisation of the core for various environments.
- The UML 2.0 Object Constraint Language: This language specifies restrictions used in diagrams.
- The UML 2.0 Diagram Interchange: It deals with the format for diagrams exchange between different tools (import/export of diagrams).

The UML language can be applied for different purposes. (Mellor, 2004) mentions the usage of the UML for the following purposes:

- UML as a sketch: The UML language can be used for drawing sketches. It is the in-formal notation of various ideas.
- The UML as a blueprint: The UML language is used for detailed design of the software. Various rules and

requirements exist for the analysis and design of the software with the usage of the UML, but concrete situation and purpose of the model decides which diagram and element of the UML will be used.

- The UML as a programming language: The UML model can be translated into the executable form. The UML can be used as a programming language. It is the most formal way of the UML usage.

Two classes of the UML 2.0 diagrams are distinguished. The static diagrams represent static structure of the investigated system. They deal with composition of crucial elements and relations between them into the structure modelling a developed system. The dynamics of the system is modelled with the usage of the diagrams representing dynamical behaviour of the system, e. g. objects interactions, lifecycle of instances of classes. Structure of the UML 2.0 is depicted in Fig. 40. Grey rectangles of the figure represent the new diagrams in the UML 2.0 in comparison to the UML 1.5. Description and explanation of each of these diagrams can be found e. g. in (Fowler, 2003), (Larman, 2004) or (Miles and Hamilton, 2006).

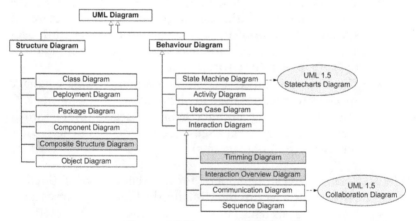

Fig. 40: UML 2.0 and diagrams

Several research studies advocate the usefulness of the UML for domain modelling of biological systems. The UML model representing protein structures is mentioned in (Bornberg-Bauer and Paton, 2002). The model is the simplification of the object-oriented data model proposed in (Gray et al., 1990) where object-oriented database system was developed for storage data about primary, secondary and tertiary protein structures. The Protein is the crucial UML class containing attributes, e. g. name, molecular weight or PDB (Protein Data Bank) code (primary identifier by which entities can be retrieved from the Protein Data Bank - repository of macromolecular structures). The aggregation (e. g. Protein consists of chains) and inheritance relationships (Helix is the SecondaryStructureElement) are used in the UML diagram between UML classes, see Fig. 41 (adjusted from ((Bornberg-Bauer and Paton, 2002), Fig. 6)).

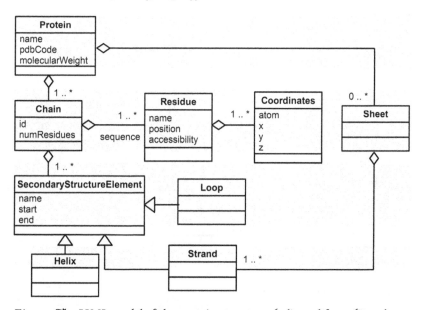

Fig. 41: The UML model of the protein structure (adjusted from (Bornberg-Bauer and Paton, 2002), Fig. 6)

The UML-based genome sequence model is proposed in (Paton et al., 2000). It represents components of eukaryotic genomes and related functional data sets. Collection of UML-based conceptual models was implemented using an object database. Basic UML class is the genome that is composed of chromosomes. Chromosomes consist of fragments - transcribed or non-transcribed regions. Fig. 42 (adjusted from (Paton et al., 2000), Fig. 1) depicts basic UML diagram for genomic data.

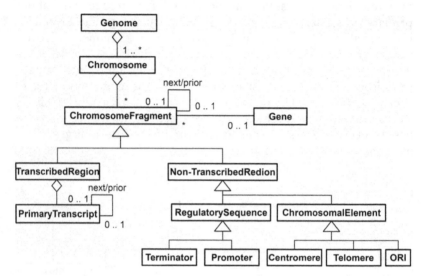

Fig. 42: Simplified UML diagram of genomic data (adjusted from (Paton et al., 2000), Fig. 1)

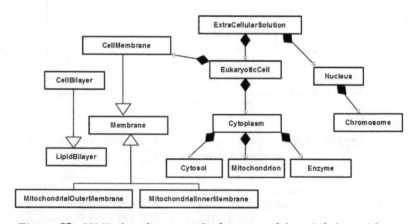

Fig. 43: The UML class diagram - the fragment of the cell (adjusted from (Webb and White, 2005), Fig. 3)

Design methodology (CellAK - Cell Assembly Kit) of cellular models is proposed in (Webb and White, 2005). It is based on five iterated steps process where the UML-based diagrams are applied for modelling of metabolic pathways (especially glycolytic pathway taking place in the cytoplasm of the cell). The CellAK process has been already used in models development and simulations of cells and cell components. Fig. 43 (adjusted from (Webb and White, 2005), Fig. 3) demonstrates the usage of the UML class diagram for modelling relations between crucial cell components.

Experimental autoimmune encephalomyelitis (EAE) is a complex autoimmune disease occurring in mice. The disease plays the role of a murine model for the multiple sclerosis in humans, because the human form of the disease shares some characteristics with the EAE. UML-based domain model of the EAE is presented in (Read et al., 2009). The UML class diagram represents static structure of the investigated system, i. e. basic entities responsible for the EAE. The UML activity diagram is used for modelling dynamic inter-cellular processes leading to the EAE or recovering from the EAE. The UML state machines diagrams represent behaviour of concrete biological entities which are important in the EAE, e. g. Th1 CD4 cells, Tc CD8 cells, Treg CD4 cells, Treg CD8 cells or dendritic cells.

Experimental Visceral Leishmaniasis (kala-azar, black fever) (EVL) is the infectious disease caused by the intra-cellular parasite of the Leishmania genus (old world (Europe, Asia, Africa) - Phlebotomus genus; new world (America, Oceania) - Lutzomyia). The disease is very serious. If the disease is untreated, the result is almost always the death of the host. The disease affects the skin, mucous membranes or organs as a bone marrow, spleen or liver. The EVL is often related with the granuloma formation process. Granuloma formation in the liver has been already modelled and simulated with the UML and agent-based approach. This process is hardly to observe directly in vivo (Flugge et al., 2009). Domain model of the granuloma formation in the EVL is mainly based on the usage of the UML class diagram, the UML state diagram and the UML sequence diagram. The UML class diagram represents basic types of biological entities occurring during the granuloma formation process. The UML state diagram models the behaviour of the T-cells, innate liver cells and macrophages (see Fig. 44, adjusted from

(Flugge et al., 2009)). The UML sequence diagram represents granuloma formation during time. The model explains why some of the granulomas are formed earlier or later. The research is in the initial stage.

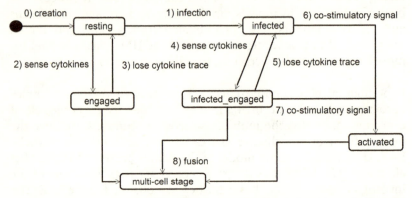

Fig. 44: States of the macrophage during granuloma formation (adjusted from (Flugge et al., 2009))

6.9   Comparison of Conceptual Approaches

The last chapter has presented a review of different approaches used for conceptual modelling of biological systems. Tab. 1 briefly summarises these approaches in chronological order (adopted, adjusted and extended from (Husáková, 2015a)). The approaches differ from each other in the level of formality and the main purpose. Concept maps are the least formal approach used for conceptualisation in the computational immunology or similar disciplines. They are primarily used for visualisation of domain-specific or general information or knowledge. Entity-relationship diagrams are not often used in computational immunology, but they are most often used in database systems development. ERD is a semi-formal language able to visualise crucial relationships between biological entities together with their most important properties. Ontologies can be viewed as informal structures used only as sketches of the investigated problem (system), but they are more often used as a formal approach for semantic web-based applications development. Bio-ontology is a special case of ontology used for modelling of bio-medical knowledge, including immunology. Statechart is a semi-formal (formal) approach focusing on modelling of the changes in states of a particular entity. They are often used for the representation of a dynamic behaviour of biological entity. The UML is mainly perceived as a semi-formal language used for analysis and design of software systems. The UML can be successfully applied in modelling of immune processes and interactions between immune cells. SBML is a markup language mainly used for formal representation of biological entities and processes occurring inside them. It is used for models sharing, similarly as the CellML formal language. CellML investigates cellular systems with the assistance of mathematical expressions and also supports models sharing. SBGN is a graphical notation able to represent different aspects of biological systems – processes, relations between biological entities and activities.

Tab. 1: Conceptual approaches in the computational imunology (adopted, adjusted and extended from (Husáková, 2015a))

ATTRIBUTE	CONCEPTUAL APPROACH	
	CONCEPT MAPS	ERD
ORIGIN	1972	1976
AUTHOR	J. D. Novak	P. Chen
ELEMENTS	concept, linking-word, cross-link	entity type relation, attribute
PURPOSE	visualisation of information and knowledge	conceptualisation of data for database systems development
USEFULNESS IN CB/CI (EXAMPLES)	concept maps for medical education	modelling of basic relations between biological entities
SOFTWARE SUPPORT	CmapTools, VUE, Visio and many others	LucidChart, Visio, SmartDraw and many others

ATTRIBUTE	CONCEPTUAL APPROACH	
	ONTOLOGIES	STATECHARTS
ORIGIN	1980	1987
AUTHOR	J. McCarthy	D. Harel
ELEMENTS	class, property, individual	state transition, action
PURPOSE	knowledge representation for communication between humans, machines or humans and machines	modelling of behaviour of reactive systems
USEFULNESS IN CB/CI (EXAMPLES)	bio-ontologies	modelling of states and transitions between states of biological entities
SOFTWARE SUPPORT	Protégé, CmapTools, Ontopia and many others	Visio, SmartDraw, AnyLogic and many others
ATTRIBUTE	CONCEPTUAL APPROACH	
	UML	SBML
ORIGIN	1996 (ver. 0.9)	2001 (Level 1)
AUTHOR	G. Booch, I. Jacobson, J. Rumbaugh	J. Doyle, H. Kitano, M. Hucka, et al.
ELEMENTS	It depends on a type of a diagram.	XML-based structure
PURPOSE	analysis and design of software systems with the UML-based diagrams	specification of machine-readable biological models
USEFULNESS IN CB/CI (EXAMPLES)	domain modelling for immune simulators development	cell signalling pathways, metabolic pathways, biochemical reactions, gene regulatory networks
SOFTWARE SUPPORT	EA, StarUML, ArgoUML and many others	Cytoscape, Biographer, CellDesigner and many others

ATTRIBUTE	CONCEPTUAL APPROACH	
	CELLML	SBGN
ORIGIN	2001 (ver. 1.0)	2005
AUTHOR	D. Bullivant, W. Hedley, P. Nielsen, et al.	H. Kitano (initiator)
ELEMENTS	XML-based structure	It depends on the language dialect: PD, ER, AF.
PURPOSE	description of cellular biological systems with the usage of mathematical expressions	unambiguous graphical notation for modelling biological systems
USEFULNESS IN CB/CI (EXAMPLES)	PD: modelling of molecular processes and changes in states of biological entities. ER: modelling of interactions and relations between biological entities, modelling of signalling pathways. AF: representation of relations between activities of biological entities.	modelling of cellular biological systems together with metadata specification for biological models (in RDF) (e. g. migration of cells, signal transduction pathways, gene regulations, etc.)
SOFTWARE SUPPORT	VirtualCell, JSim, OpenCell and many others	CellDesigner, Athena, Arcadia and many others

7. Agent Modelling Language for Computational Immunology

The AML (Agent Modelling Language) is an UML-based semi-formal visual language used to model systems in terms of concepts applied in multi-agent systems (MAS). The reason for specification of a new conceptual language is that the traditional modelling languages used in software engineering are not suitable for modelling of agent and multi-agent systems. The AML is based on the UML 2.0 Superstructure describing particular diagrams in the view of abstract syntax, semantics and UML notation. The AML is useful for modelling of systems (Cervenka et al., 2006):

- composed of autonomous, concurrent and asynchronous entities,
- containing entities able to (pro-actively) interact with each other and the environment,
- where entities are able to offer or use services,
- that enable the fulfilling of goals and decomposition of (complex) solved problems,
- containing entities with the ability to use their mental characteristic for decision making.

The AML meta-model is composed of five packages (Cervenka and Trencansky, 2007). Each of them is focused on the modelling of specific aspects of the investigated system:

- Architecture: The package contains elements for modelling entity types of the multi-agent system (agent type, resource type, environment type), MAS deployment and social aspects related to the behaviour of the agent types (role types, roles playing, social associations).
- Mental: The package contains elements for representation of mental states (believes, goals, plans and mental relationships).
- Behaviours: The package offers elements for the modelling of basic behaviours of agents (behaviour decomposition, observations and effecting interactions, services), mobility and communicative interactions).
- Ontologies: The package contains elements for representation of ontologies (classes, relations, merging or importing).
- Model management: The package is focused on situation-based modelling for contextual information representation.

7.1 CATEGORISATION OF DIAGRAMS

The AML offers eleven diagrams extending the UML, see Fig. 46. The new categorisation of the AML diagrams is proposed in the monograph, see Fig. 45. The new groups of the AML diagrams are specified on the basis of their similar properties and use. The first group comprises diagrams modelling the internal architecture of the entity type (agent types, resource types and environment types). These AML diagrams focus on agent-based architectures (sensors, effectors, internal services, behaviour of each agent, mental attitudes, goals or plans). The second group contains diagrams used for representation of the external architecture of the investigated system – the multi-agent system. This collection of diagrams is separated into three subgroups. Basic relations between entity types together with their social organisation are a part of the static view. Interactions between entity types are modelled with the AML sequence diagrams and AML communication diagrams in the dynamic view. MAS deployment is a part of the physical view. Context view exists between these two groups of the AML diagrams, because it is related with each of them. Fig. 46 depicts the classification of the AML diagrams. The following paragraph will describe briefly the AML diagrams.

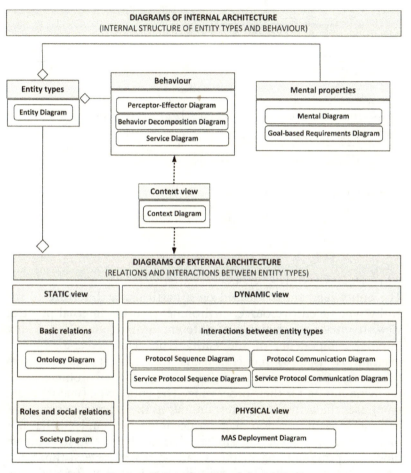

Fig. 45: Proposed classification of the AML diagrams

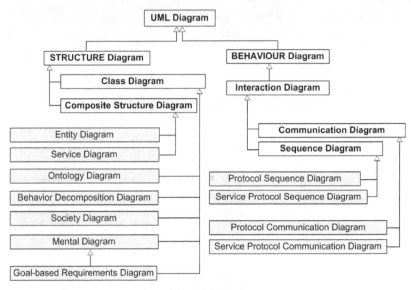

Fig. 46: The AML diagrams

7.1.1   Diagrams of the internal architecture

The entity diagram is focused on a particular architecture of the entity type (agent, resource, environment) in the internal point of view. It integrates elements of different AML diagrams modelling internal components of the entity type. The perceptor-effector diagram is used to model sensors (perceptors) and actuators (effectors). Sensors are used for sensing the environment and receiving inputs for their processing. The entity type (mainly agent type) uses the actuators for responding to the external stimuli. The behaviour decomposition diagram decomposes complex behaviour into simpler parts sharing similar characteristics. These compact blocks of programming methods can be reused several times and executed concurrently. The service diagram is applied for modelling of services offered/used by the entity types. The service can be represented from the internal or the external point of view. Internal components (modules) of the entity type can use internal services which are offered/used by internal components from the internal point of view. The service can be offered/used by the entity type as a whole from the external point of view. The mental diagram represents believes, plans, goals and mental relations of entity types. The goal-based requirements diagram is mainly applied for modelling of relations between goals. Fig. 47 depicts a graphical representation of crucial AML-based elements used for modelling of internal architecture of the entity type with the AML.

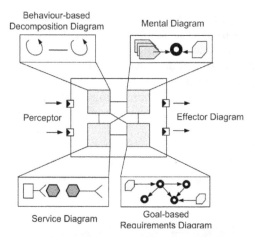

Fig. 47: AML-based diagrams of the internal architecture

7.1.2 DIAGRAMS OF THE EXTERNAL ARCHITECTURE

An entity diagram is one of the most important AML diagrams. It offers a basic overview of the external structure of a multi-agent system. It is based on three entity types: an agent type, a resource type and an environment type. The agent type represents classes of agents - intelligent entities able to solve autonomously a particular task. The environment type specifies the surrounding environment (conditions for existence) where the agent types "live". The environment is also perceived as the autonomous entity. The resource type plays the role of a behavioural entity representing the source that is used by the agent types or environment types to fulfil their goals. The information or knowledge source is a typical example of the resource type. An ontology diagram is used for the modelling of simple ontological hierarchies. This diagram is not suitable for modelling complex ontologies with expression of their semantics. Different tools are more appropriate for representation of formal ontologies, e. g. Protégé or TopBraid Composer. A society diagram highlights social relations between entity types (an agent type, a resource type, an environment type). It is able to represent organisation units, social roles and peer-to-peer or super-ordinate/sub-ordinate social relations between entity types. Interactions and their protocols are modelled with the sequence and communication diagrams. A protocol sequence diagram is used for modelling of interaction protocols. A service protocol sequence diagram is applied in modelling of service protocols. A protocol communication diagram focuses on modelling of interaction protocols in terms of the communication diagrams. A service protocol communication diagram represents service protocols. A MAS deployment diagram is used for representation of deployment activity of MAS into physical environment. Fig. 48 depicts graphical representation of crucial AML-based elements used for modelling of external architecture of the entity type with the AML.

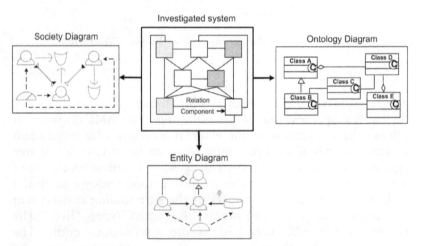

Fig. 48: AML-based diagrams of the external architecture

7.2 SOFTWARE SUPPORT

The StarUML is an open-source software primarily used for design and analysis of software systems with the application of the UML 2.0 (StarUML [n. d.]). Its functionality can be extended by plugins. The StarUML 5 can integrate the AML plugin based on the specification of the AML language (Cervenka and Trencansky, 2007) for modelling of multi-agent systems. It would appear that the StarUML 5 is the only freely available software supporting the AML (in time of monograph writing). This is why this product is used in the following case study, see the chapter 8, where conceptual modelling of specific immune processes with the AML is investigated. Tab. 2 mentions AML diagrams and corresponding toolboxes in the StarUML. Fig. 49 offers a picture of the StarUML environment together with the proposed structure of packages with AML diagrams.

Tab. 2: AML diagrams and StarUML toolboxes

AML DIAGRAM	StarUML TOOLBOX
Entity diagram	(AML) Architecture (AML) Behavior (AML) Mental
Perceptor-effector diagram	(AML) Behavior
Service diagram	(AML) Behavior
Mental diagram	(AML) Mental
Goal-based requirements diagram	(AML) Mental
Ontology diagram	(AML) Ontology
Society diagram	(AML) Architecture
Protocol sequence diagram	(AML) Communicative Sequence diagram
Service protocol sequence diagram	(AML) Communicative Sequence Role diagram
Protocol communication diagram	(AML) Communicative Collaboration diagram
Service protocol communication diagram	(AML) Communicative Collaboration Role diagram
MAS deployment diagram	(AML) MAS Deployment

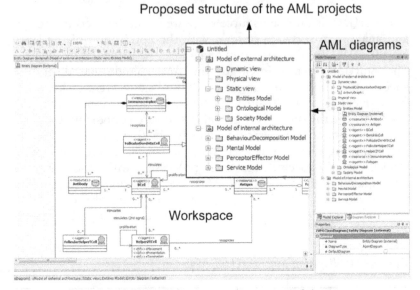

Fig. 49: *The StarUML and the proposed structure of the AML projects*

8. CASE STUDY

The lymphatic system consists of compact and complex units – lymph nodes. Lymph node is a secondary lymphoid organ offering a place where the "fight" between immune cells and "enemies" occurs and where the adaptive immunity is initiated (Abbas et al., 2011). Research in trafficking of cells of the innate and adaptive immunity through this lymphoid organ is very important because it can help better understanding of the immune cells influence on each other and their contribution to the maintenance of homeostasis in the lymph node. The AML language is applied in order to demonstrate its usefulness for modelling of processes occurring in the lymph node.

The following section looks at the description of lymph node architecture and the processes occurring inside this complex structure. Attention is mainly aimed at the processes occurring in the paracortex of the lymph node, especially the behaviour of naive T-cells and dendritic cells, together with interactions between them. AML diagrams are mentioned and focused on the modelling of the key players and processes occurring in the paracortex of the lymph node of the mouse in a non-inflammatory state.

8.1 LYMPH NODE – FUNCTION AND ARCHITECTURE

The lymph node is a secondary lymphoid organ playing the role of filtration system where immune cells (especially macrophages and dendritic cells) monitor the lymph flow in the lymph node and collect antigens from the flow. The lymph is a fluid circulating in the lymphatic system. It contains potentially dangerous antigens which can be detected by various immune cells. The lymph node is the environment where the naive lymphocytes (B-cells, T-cells) can be activated on the basis of recognition of antigenic peptides presented by antigen-presenting cells (APC) (e. g. dendritic cells). These immune cells become the effector mature cells and monitor the environment outside the lymph node where the potential danger can occur.

The lymph node is a complex and dynamic three-dimensional structure composed of three layers, see Fig. 50 (adopted and adjusted from (Husáková, 2014)). Each of them consists of specific immune cells maintaining homeostasis in the lymph node. The cortex (B-cell area) is a place where a high concentration of B-cells and follicular dendritic cells (FDC) occurs (Abbas et al., 2011). B-cells play the role of plasmatic or memory cells and cells interacting with the follicular dendritic cells (FDC). The FDCs present intact antigens to B-cells and are involved in the development and maintenance of a stromal network helping with the movement of B-cells in the B-cell area. They are producers of chemokines influencing the trafficking of B-cells in the cortex. Paracortex (T-cell area) is a place where a high concentration of T-cells, dendritic cells and fibroblastic reticular cells (FRC) occurs. This location is the main area of the lymph node where the interaction between naive T-cells and dendritic cells occur. Naive T-cells can be stimulated by dendritic cells presenting antigenic peptides to naive T-cells. They can eliminate antigens, regulate different immune functions or stimulate immune cells. FRCs are fibroblastic reticular cells producing collagen-rich reticular fibres and form a stromal network. This network helps with the movement of immune cells in the paracortex, similar to the case of the network produced by FDCs in the cortex. FRCs release chemokines influencing movement of the cells in the paracortex. Medulla mainly contains phagocytic cells – macrophages. These cells present antigens to T-cells and B-cells, and eliminate dangerous antigens with phagocytosis. Medullary reticular network occurs also in the medulla.

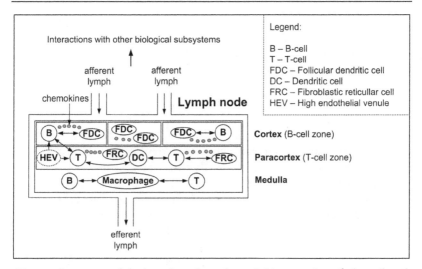

Fig. 50: Structure of the lymph node and crucial interactions (adopted and adjusted from (Husáková, 2014))

8.2 KEY STEPS OF MIGRATION OF T-CELLS IN THE LYMPH NODE

The T-cell is perceived as a mobile autonomous entity of which there are two types. The CD4+ T-cell specialises as a helper T-cell after the contact with a cognate antigen in the lymph node. The CD8+ T-cell specialises as form of the cytotoxic T-cell after the contact with a cognate antigen. For simplicity, these two types of T-cells are not going to be distinguished here. Naive T-cells can start to migrate into the lymph node through two entry points: the afferent lymph or the high endothelial venules (HEV). Only a fraction of naive T-cells enters the lymph node with the aid of afferent lymph. The migration through the HEV is described as a multistep adhesion cascade. More details about this process can be found e. g. in (von Andrian and Mempel, 2003) or (Girard et al., 2012).

Intra-nodal migration and positioning is the second phase of the naive T-cell migration. Most studies describe migration as a random process (Miller et al., 2002), (Wei et al., 2003), (Miller et al., 2004). (Bajenoff et al., 2006) justifies the view of migration as random and predictable thanks to the existence of the FRC network. The same study also mentions that naive T-cells are in contact with the reticular fibres of the FRC network immediately after leaving the HEV. According to (Wei et al., 2003), collisions between lymphocytes do not have noticeable effect on the movement of other cells. T-cells do not perceive the FRC network and their reticular fibres as a barrier. They actively follow these fibres. In some rare cases, T-cells jumped between neighbouring fibres. Similar results about deterministic movement of T-cells in the FRC network are mentioned e. g. in (Beltman et al., 2007). The most recent study advocates the influence of the FRC network on the direction of movement of T-cells. CCL19 chemokine and CCL21 chemokine (produced by the FRC) influence the speed of migration in the FRC network (Worbs et al., 2007), (Okada and Cyster, 2007).

Egress from the lymph node is the third phase of the naive T-cell migration. If the naive T-cell is activated, it differentiates, proliferates and migrates to the medulla and through the efferent lymph towards the locations where the inflammation is taking place. If the naive T-cell is not activated during some time, it migrates through the medulla and efferent lymph and tries to enter to the other lymph node. The process of egressing is a complex process. It is influenced by the chemo-attractant S1P (Spingosine-1-phosphate) occurring in the blood or lymph (Abbas et al., 2011). S1P is released by many types of cell types. S1P is released by lymphatic endothelial cells which are in the inner side of the cortical sinuses (Cyster and Schwab, 2012) (blind-ended lymphatic vessels located in the T-cell areas of the lymph nodes mediating exit of the B-cells and T-cells from the lymph nodes).

8.3   Key players occurring in the paracortex

The roles and characteristics of T-cells in the lymph node are described in the subchapter 8.2. A fibre reticular cell (FRC) is the second entity playing important role in trafficking of immune cells. FRCs are producers of reticular fibres forming stromal reticular network. This network offers pathways for movement of immune cells occurring in the paracortex (especially for T-cells and dendritic cells) (Katakai et al., 2004). It directs lymphocytes towards the antigen-presenting cells, especially dendritic cells offering antigens to T-cells. FRCs reside on these fibres and release chemotactic products – especially chemokines CCL19, CCL21 "attracting" the immune cells. It is not clear how the fibres are changed during inflammation. (Katakai et al., 2004) mentions that the reticular network is dramatically reorganised during the immune response. Dendritic cell (DC) is the third entity playing an important role in the paracortex and influencing the T-cells. Dendritic cell is a professional antigen presenting cell and phagocytic cell. Majority of DCs enter to the lymph node through the afferent lymph towards the HEV areas where they reside and wait for naive T-cells for presenting antigens and activation of naive T-cells. Two models describing interactions between DC and naive T-cells exist at present (Cahalan and Parker, 2005), (Henrickson and von Andrian, 2007):

1. Stable interaction model is based on the forming of immunological synapses between naive T-cells and DCs. This process is initiated by interactions between adhesion molecules of the naive T-cells and antigen-presenting cells.
2. Serial encounter model (stochastic) is based on short-lasting contacts between DCs and naive T-cells until the naive T-cells receive enough contacts for their activation.

The second model is favoured for conceptual modelling of basic interactions between DCs and T-cells.

8.4   EXTERNAL ARCHITECTURE - STATIC VIEW

8.4.1 ONTOLOGY DIAGRAM

The ontology diagram highlights hierarchical relations between the most important "players" for the maintenance of homeostasis in the lymph node, see Fig. 51. The pluripotent hematopoietic stem cell is the most general ontological class. This type of cell is then specialised into the common myeloid or lymphoid progenitor. As you can see, not all descendants are included in the ontology diagram (e. g. neutrophils, basophils or mast cells). Only the most important immune cells with direct relation to the lymph node are modelled by the ontology diagram. A connective tissue cell, an organ and a tissue are distinguished as the most general ontological classes in the second part of the ontology diagram. It is obvious that the primary lymphoid organs (a bone marrow and a thymus) exist, but the abstraction is used for the integration of the key biological entities in concept modelling of the events occurring in the lymph node.

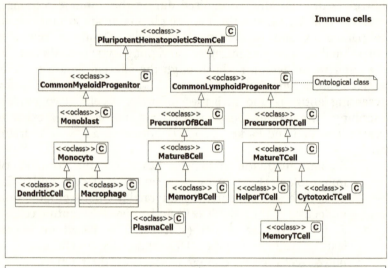

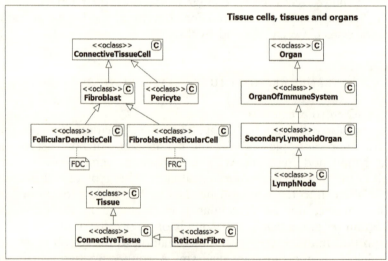

Fig. 51: External architecture (static view) - Ontology diagram

8.4.2 ENTITY DIAGRAM

The entity diagram emphasises the key entity types occurring in all layers of the lymph node. The main attention is paid to the relations occurring between entity types in the paracortex of the lymph node. The lymph node is represented as the environment where interactions between B-cells, T-cells, dendritic cells and macrophages occur. All types of relations (an association, an aggregation, a composition, an inheritance) used in the UML can be applied also in the entity diagram. The entity diagram distinguishes between agent types and resource types. The agent type is the autonomous entity following specific goal. The immune cells or pathogens are represented as agent types. The AML does not offer entity for representation of structures. Structure type is proposed as the new AML element in the monograph. The structure type is defined as the non-autonomous entity created with the use of resource types or agent types and marked by stereotype <<structure>>. A stromal network consisting of reticular fibres is perceived as the structure type, see Fig. 52.

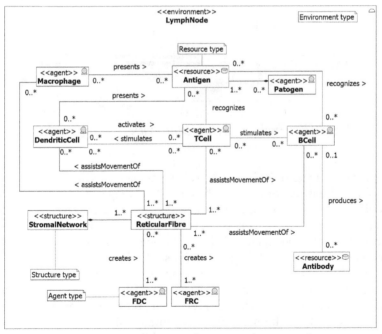

Fig. 52: External architecture (static view) - Entity diagram

8.4.3 SOCIETY DIAGRAM

The society diagram emphasises social roles played by entity types. Fig. 53 represents structural relations between entity types and social roles. As the example, the fibre reticular cell (FDC) and the follicular dendritic cell (FDC) play the role of the reticular fibre producer. The producer of the reticular fibre is represented as the social role. Lymph node is a layered system consisting of the paracortex, the cortex and the medulla (for more details, see the subchapter 8.1.). These layers are represented as organisation unit types of the lymph node.

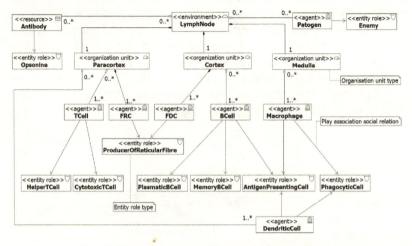

Fig. 53: External architecture (static view) - Society diagram

Fig. 54 represents only social roles and social relations between biological entities of the lymph node. This diagram emphasises the social relations existing between crucial social roles. As the example, the $T_{cytotoxic}$-cell is able to eliminate the enemy – the pathogen (the antigen). The peer-to-peer social relation exists between these two biological entities. Producer of reticular fibres offer the pathways for movement of immune cells. Super-ordinate/sub-ordinate social relation exists between these two social roles because the producer of reticular fibres probably fundamentally influences the movement of immune cells and specifies conditions for the trafficking of immune cells.

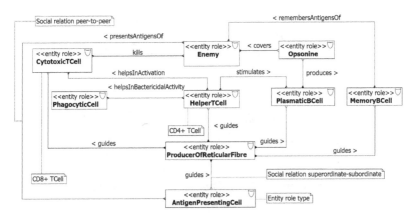

Fig. 54: External architecture (static view) - Social relations

8.5 EXTERNAL ARCHITECTURE - DYNAMIC VIEW

8.5.1 PROTOCOL COMMUNICATION DIAGRAM

The protocol communication diagram is a special case of the UML communication diagram. It models the information stream between entity types where the order of communication messages is important. The AML-based communication diagram uses the notation of the UML-based communication diagram. It includes the entity types (or social roles) and interactions between them in a particular order. Fig. 55 depicts interactions between T-cells, dendritic cells and reticular fibres. The order of interactions is highlighted by numbers. Interaction is specified by its name corresponding to the intended method of the AML-based class. Arguments are not mentioned in these methods, because the AML-based diagrams are focused on domain modelling. They are not focused on platform modelling (see the CoSMoS process in the chapter 5). The AML-based communication diagram is simplified because parallel interactions are not included in the diagram and it cannot be said that the order of interactions is the same under different conditions.

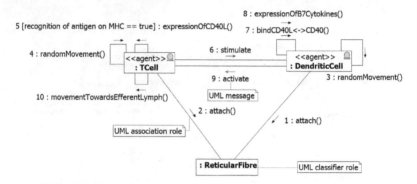

Fig. 55: External architecture (dynamic view) - interactions between T-cells and dendritic cells

8.6 Internal architecture – behaviour

8.6.1 Perceptor-effector diagram

The perceptor-effector diagram is useful for representation of surface molecules of immune cells. Surface structures play the role of perceptors or effectors. Fig. 56 depicts roles of surface molecules in case of the T-cells, dendritic cells and B-cells. The diagram represents the roles of chemokines produced by reticular cells (FRC, FDC) and their influence on the behaviour of the immune cells (T-cells, dendritic cells and B-cells). The diagram points out only some of the chemokines influencing the movement of immune cells. Not all of them are considered and represented in the diagram. As an example, the fibre reticular cell (FRC) is the producer of the chemokines CCL19 and CCL21. These ones are represented as resources – information messengers. These two chemokines are perceived by T-cells (the receptor CCR7), dendritic cells (the receptor CCR7) and B-cell (the receptor CCR7).

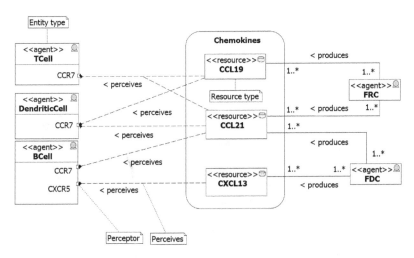

Fig. 56: Internal architecture (behaviour) - crucial interactions in the stromal network

Fig. 57 represents a different situation. It represents possible interactions between T-cells and dendritic cells leading to the activation (proliferation and differentiation) of the T-cells with the assistance of cytokines. The diagram can be described as follows (Abbas and Lichtman, 2010): The dendritic cell presents antigenic peptides with the MHC-I (for CD8+ T-cells) or with the MHC-II (for CD4+ T-cells). These two surface structures and immune cell types are not distinguished in the perceptor-effector diagram. Antigens are perceived by the T-cell with the TCR – the T-cell receptor. This event causes the expression of the CD40L on the surface of the T-cell. CD40L binds to the CD40 – surface molecule presented on the dendritic cell. This event leads to the expression of the B7 molecule and secretion of the cytokines by the dendritic cell. These cytokines stimulate the T-cell for proliferation and differentiation with the assistance of other cytokines, e. g. interleukins IL-1 and IL-12.

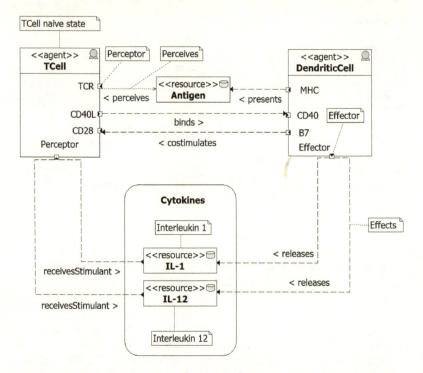

Fig. 57: Internal architecture (behaviour) - interactions between T-cells and dendritic cells

8.6.2 BEHAVIOUR-BASED DECOMPOSITION DIAGRAM

The behaviour-based decomposition diagram models the behaviour of the entity type with the help of behaviour fragments. Behaviour fragments are compact units consisting of operations sharing similar characteristics. These blocks of operations can be reused by various entity types. Fig. 58 depicts the definition and application of behaviour fragments for the dendritic cell. Four behaviour fragments are distinguished:

- AntigenPresentation: The fragment collects operations related to the presentation of antigens on the surface of the dendritic cell.
- Recognition: Recognition of surrounding particles is one of the most important abilities of immune cells. It depends on the bind between the cell and the "foreign" particle. This

behaviour fragment is a part of the AntigenPresentation fragment because the presentation of antigens requires recognition of antigens.

- CellDeath: Only two ways of cell death are distinguished – apoptosis (programmed cell death) and necrosis (abnormal and harmful cause of the cell death).
- Movement: The fragment collects operations related to the movement of the dendritic cell. Only two operations are considered – following of the reticular fibres of the stromal network and detection of barriers.

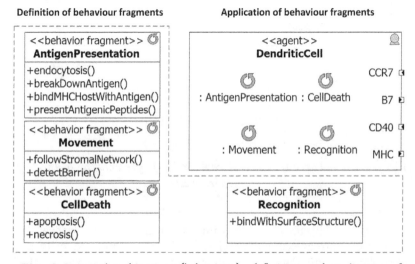

Fig. 58: Internal architecture (behaviour) - definition and application of behaviour fragments

8.6.3 SERVICE(S) DIAGRAM

The service diagram represents services used by/offered by the entity types. Fig. 59 depicts the simplified internal structure of the dendritic cell. Integral parts of the dendritic cell use or offer services. Only basic subsystems of the dendritic cells relating with the antigen internalization are represented in the service diagram. For example, dendritic cell binds the antigen with the assistance of the MHC (the sensor). Antigen fragmentation is one of the most important internal services "offered by" the lysosome and "used by" the host MHC. This service is responsible for division antigens into the smaller fragments which are presented on the surface of the dendritic cell with the assistance of the MHC (the effector). These antigenic peptides are recognised e. g. by the T-cells.

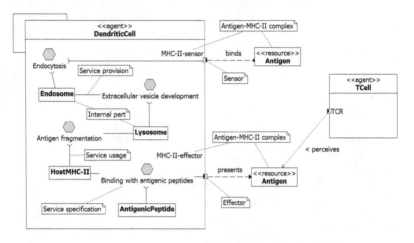

Fig. 59: Internal architecture (internal services) - presentation of antigens by dendritic cells

The service diagram represents internal and external services. Fig. 60 depicts three external services. Follicular dendritic cells and fibroblastic reticular cells offer the external service called <Production of reticular fibre>. This external service is used by the immune cell for movement. Dendritic cell offers the external service called <Antigen presentation> used by the T-cells or B-cells. T$_{helper}$-cell offers the external service called <Stimulation> used by the B-cell. Internal and external services can be a part of one service diagram. These services are separated in this case study because of the readability of the service diagram.

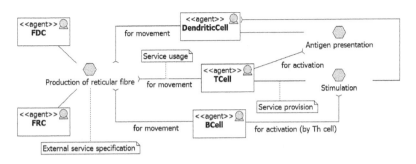

Fig. 60: Internal architecture (external services) - basic view

8.6.4 MENTAL DIAGRAM

The mental diagram models mental attitudes of autonomous entity types. It is used for representation of goals, believes, plans, mental relationships (contributions, responsibilities), mental actions (committing or cancellation of goals) and mental constraints. At the first sight, it does not make sense to model mental characteristics for the immune cells. Mental attitudes are typical for humans, not for cells. On the other hand, a cell can be perceived as a socially autonomous entity living in communities and having mental dispositions which are used for goals fulfilment or following some plans (Walker et al., 2004), (Smallwood and Holcombe, 2006). Mental models of biological systems can be valuable for modelling plausible models of the NIS or for the investigation of similarities and differences among social life of cells and humans. A simplified mental diagram of the dendritic cell is depicted on Fig. 61. The dendritic cell has four plans: presentation of intracellular products, presentation of extracellular products, co-stimulation of immune cells and binding with CD40 ligand. These plans are supported by believes that the dendritic cell can follow these plans and fulfil goals that are part of these plans. Responsibility for goals can be defined with the help of the mental relationship responsibility.

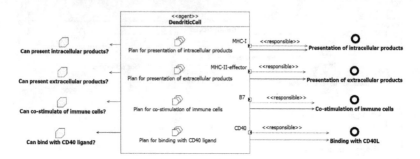

Fig. 61: Internal architecture - mental diagram for dendritic cell

9. CONTRIBUTIVENESS OF AGENT MODELLING LANGUAGE

The chapter 8 presents the application of the Agent Modelling Language for representation of the immune cells trafficking through the secondary lymphoid organ – the lymph node. The main attention is paid to the representation of interactions between white blood cells – T-cells and dendritic cells. The multi-agent system is the natural alternative for modelling complexity of the natural immune system. It uses the concept of an intelligent agent dealing autonomously during problem solving. It is able to coordinate and co-operate its activities with other intelligent agents and form communities for collective goals fulfilment. Immune cells share similar characteristics with intelligent agents where agents can play the role of templates for representation of immune cells. The Agent Modelling Language is a promising approach for analysis and design of systems simulating behaviour of particular aspects of the natural immune system. This language is beneficial only if the entities of the natural immune system are modelled in terms of the multi-agent systems (Husáková, 2015b). The AML is more precise in several aspects of the natural immune system modelling in comparison to the UML. The usefulness of the AML-based diagrams is described below where the most useful AML-based diagrams are mentioned together with their characteristics and elements beneficial for modelling of the natural immune system:

- The ontology diagram (the UML class diagram): The UML class diagram can be used instead of the ontology diagram if it is not necessary to use terms of ontological engineering for modelling. The UML class diagram is sufficient for modelling structural and hierarchical aspects of the natural immune system. The ontology diagram can use the same relations (an association, an aggregation, a composition, an inheritance) as the UML class diagram. The ontology diagram can represent only elementary ontologies and ontological classes without semantic descriptions or definitions of classes. The RDF(S) or the OWL language is the more efficient approach for modelling of ontologies.

    o   Useful elements: an ontology class

- The entity diagram (the UML class diagram): The entity diagram distinguishes three entity types (an agent type, a resource type, an environment type) that can be applied for modelling of biological entities. The new structural entity type <<structure>> is proposed in the case study (see the chapter 8). The entity diagram structures conceptual views on the reality in terms of the MAS. The UML language does not deal with an agent, a resource and an environment, but these ones are modelled as the UML classes.

    o   Useful elements: an agent type, an environment type, a resource type

- The society diagram (the UML class diagram): The society diagram models social aspects of the biological system. It integrates social roles, social relationships (peer-to-peer, super-ordinate/sub-ordinate, play association) and organisation unit types consisting of social roles and social relations. This diagram is useful if the social behaviour can be detected in the natural immune system, e. g. in case of the interactions between immune cells. Pro-social (cooperative) and competitive behaviour is visible in the natural immune system. Normal white cells are able to cooperate and coordinate towards maintenance of homeostasis. They are able to undergo apoptosis for elimination inadequate behaviour. Abnormal cells (e. g. cancer cells) have antisocial behaviour. They can occupy territory and defend own interests against interests of the normal cells. They can influence behaviour of the normal cells against the organism.

    o   Useful elements: an organisation unit type, an entity role type, a social association, a play association

- The service diagram (the UML composite structure diagram): The service diagram models abilities (services) of biological systems, i. e. what these systems can offer (a service provision dependency) and use (a service usage dependency). Services can be represented as internal and external. Internal services are offered or used by internal components of the entity type. External services are offered or used by entity types as compact units. The UML deals with the services, especially web services.

    o   Useful elements: a service specification, a service provision, a dependency, a service usage

- The perceptor-effector diagram (the UML class diagram): The perceptor-effector diagram models sensing and effecting interactions of entity types. The diagram is useful in case of representation of the surface molecules of the immune cells. The diagram models static aspects of the investigated system, but it can visualise "interactions" between entity types – what the immune cell uses for receiving inputs from the environment and what the immune cell uses for reactions on these stimuli. The UML does not offer these characteristics, but perceptors and effectors are represented as UML ports.

    o   Useful elements: a perceptor (+ a type), an effector (+ a type), a perceives dependency, an effects dependency

- The behaviour-based decomposition diagram (the UML class diagram): The behaviour-based decomposition diagram uses behaviour fragments – abstract concepts representing similar operations in one compact unit called behaviour fragment. It is the UML class and it can use the same relationships as in case of the UML class diagram. This diagram is useful only if we can find more operations sharing similar characteristics of the entity type. It is not completely necessary to use these behaviour fragments, as they are related rather with the specification of the platform model (see the chapter 5).

- o   Useful elements: a behaviour fragment, a behaviour fragment property
- The mental diagram (the UML class diagram): The mental diagram is useful if biological entities are represented as systems having mental states (believes, goals, plans). The individual cell does not have mental characteristics similar to humans. Behaviour of a cell is encoded in the DNA (the deoxyribonucleic acid). On the other hand, a cell behaves like a social entity, because it lives in communities, displays competitive or pro-social behaviour and tries to fulfil goals prescribed by the DNA. Mental models of biological entities can be useful for a development of plausible models of the NIS behaviour or for an investigation of similarities and differences between the social life of cells and humans (Husáková, 2015). Relations between entity types and mental states are represented by mental associations or mental responsibilities. Mental states are not offered by the UML, but they are represented as UML classes.
- The protocol communication diagram (the UML communication diagram): The protocol communication diagram represents interactions among entity types (social roles) in a particular order. Entity types (social roles) play the role of "messengers" transmitting communication messages. Relations between "messengers" are modelled as the UML association roles, but the UML message is particular communication message. There are few differences in comparison to the UML-based communication diagram. The AML-based communication diagram includes entity types or social roles as interacting parties of the diagram. It can represent changes of social roles (create/destroy attribute). This aspect is not modelled in the diagram, see Fig. 55. The diagram is useful only if small amount of interaction is considered.
  - o   Useful elements: a create attribute, a destroy attribute, a multi-message, a join subset

The following Tab. 3 summarises the usefulness of the AML-based diagrams for the conceptual domain modelling in computational immunology. The first eight AML diagrams were tested for the use in computational immunology. The next six AML diagrams were not tested, but their use has been proposed and advocated. Only the most useful AML diagrams have the tick sign in the Tab. 3. This table is based on a personal experience with these diagrams in the case study presented (see the chapter 8).

Tab. 3: Usefulness of the AML in the computational immunology

AML DIAGRAM	APPLICATION IN THE CI
Ontology diagram	×
Entity diagram	✓
Society diagram	✓
Service diagram	✓
Perceptor-effector diagram	✓
Behaviour-based decomposition diagram	×
Mental diagram	✓
Protocol communication diagram	✓
Protocol sequence diagram	✓
Service protocol sequence diagram	✓
Service protocol communication diagram	✓
Goal-based requirements diagram	×
MAS deployment diagram	×
Context diagram	✓

Several AML-based diagrams are not used in the case study focusing on the conceptualisation of processes occurring in the lymph node. The protocol sequence diagram and the service sequence diagram are special cases of the UML sequence diagram. These AML-based interactions diagrams represent interaction protocols and service protocols with the UML-based sequence diagrams notation. Diagrams can integrate interactions between entity types or social roles without the necessity to mention the order of messages in comparison to the communication diagram. Diagrams are suitable for modelling of more complex interactions between interested parties. The service communication diagram is based on the UML communication diagram, but it offers elements for services representation. It is considered that these diagrams can be useful for computational immunology, similar to the protocol communication diagram. The goal-based requirements diagram is a special case of the mental diagram. It focuses on the modelling of business goals captured by means of elements in the mental diagram. It can be used also for modelling of functional or non-functional requirements during analysis of a software application (Cervenka and Trencansky, 2007). The MAS deployment diagram is used for representation of physical infrastructure of the developed multi-agent system. Physical infrastructure plays the role of the agent execution environment. The main attention is paid to the domain modelling of particular immune processes. The deployment of the MAS is not considered. Situation-based modelling is used for context representation. The investigated system is modelled in the view of various situations that can happen and influence its behaviour. Each situation is represented by a particular AML-based diagram or a combination of them that are part of the context (the package). The complete model consists of all contexts (packages). The context diagram could be useful for modelling of complex systems dealing with various situations.

10. CONCLUSION

The difficulties facing computer immunology-based research are obvious. The natural immune system is very complex system consisting of many "players" interacting with each other. Many feedback loops and interconnections of the natural immune system with other systems cause the natural immune system to be hard to investigate and understand. Also, some facts about the behaviour of the natural immune system are missing, because it is difficult to explore the particular process in vivo or in vitro. Technologies that could be able to measure some specific parameters, have not yet been developed. Put differently, immunologists have not yet suggested how to measure and collect such data. These are the reasons why the natural immune system is difficult to model and simulate. Computational immunology proposes the use of in silico approaches where a combination of "immunological expertise", methods of computer science, mathematics, physics and statistics can help with answering questions related to serious diseases, and improve the quality of life. Research in the field of computational immunology is not easy, because it presupposes a multi-disciplinary approach. The complexity of the natural immune system is not a challenge only for computer scientists, mathematicians, physicists or statisticians, but often also for medical doctors, biologists or chemists. Complexity of the natural immune system is one of the reasons why computer scientists do not pay enough attention to computational immunology. From the beginning, it is the most difficult to distinguish which properties or mechanisms of immunity are more and which are less important for non-experts in immunology. An expert input is necessary because it can help to avoid misunderstandings which could end up making their way into the model. An expert can help them to recognise which level of abstraction is appropriate for a particular case. On the other hand, the "modellers" should posses some background information concerning the behaviour of the natural immune system, as this will make the information or knowledge supplied by the expert more acceptable and simpler. The "modeller" will be able to ask the right questions. Missing feedback and discussion with experts can integrate uncertainty into the model. Then the model would be based on wrong assumptions. The social dimension of computational immunology-based research is also obvious, but not only in this research area. It can also be a challenge to persuade immunologists that the developed models and simulations can be useful and they can be useful, and can bring added value to the understanding of the application domain.

Immunology is a fast growing discipline. It is necessary to use the most current information sources for models development since immunological papers published four or five years ago do not, in most cases, offer the most up to date information about the state of the research. Abstraction and parameters estimation is inevitable, but the aim is to model towards faithful models that should be reflective of the real biological system. Success in the investigation of immunity with in silico approaches is based on teamwork, the bringing together of various people with different kinds of knowledge in order to study the amazing complexity of the natural immune system. The natural immune system is an inspiration for solving all kinds of problems. This monograph has introduced artificial immune systems as adaptive systems. They integrate selected immune principles into algorithms that can help to solve, or improve solutions of problems in computer science, optimization, engineering, data analysis, planning or scheduling. A "killer application" for which the immune algorithms can be applied as the best solution has not yet been clearly defined. Immune algorithms are promising solutions for problems where the stability and robustness are crucial properties of the system. The complexity of the natural immune systems can be investigated by in vitro, in vivo or in silico approaches. Computational immunology offers in silico approaches helping with the understanding of phenomena that are difficult to explore through traditional techniques. The main aim of this area is to investigate in detail the relations between components of the natural immune system and complex interactions between them. This activity could help to improve vaccine development, to support efficiency of drugs or receive more accurate predictions of behaviour of the natural immune system. This monograph has introduced the historical context of computational immunology and the first computer science-based applications. Various conceptual modelling approaches are proposed for the representation of the most important biological entities and interactions. They differ from each other in the degree of formality and use. Concept maps are informal graphical structures together with the entity-relationship diagrams. XML-based languages – SBML and CellML are machine-readable formats able to represent cellular and other biological systems, and offer the structure for models sharing. The UML is a semi-formal standardised language useful for domain modelling in computational immunology. The UML class diagram, the UML state-machine diagram and the UML activity diagram are mainly used for conceptualisation of immune processes. Statecharts are semi-formal (formal) approach for description of discrete behaviour of the investigated system. Statecharts are used in modelling changes in states of the biological entities. Ontologies play various roles in knowledge representation. According to (Roussey et al., 2011), ontologies can be used as informal structures depicting information or knowledge as a sketch. Formal ontologies are used for building knowledge bases of intelligent agents, reasoning and building applications of the semantic web.

The AML language is an extension of the UML used for multi-agent systems analysis and development. The AML is investigated in detail in this monograph - in the view of conceptualisation of processes occurring in the natural immune system. Eight AML-based diagrams are used for domain modelling of processes occurring in the secondary lymphoid organ – the lymph node where interactions between T-cells and dendritic cells are mainly taken into account. It is found out that the following tested AML diagrams are useful for domain modelling in the computational immunology: the entity diagram, the society diagram, the protocol communication diagram, the perceptor-effector diagram, the service diagram and the mental diagram. The entity diagram is useful for visualisation of the most important biological entities and relations between them. It is similar to the UML class diagram, but the entity diagram deals with agent types existing in the MAS. The society diagram is also similar to the UML class diagram, but it emphasises social relationships between entity types and social roles. Social relationships can be represented also in case of the artificial immune system where immune cells play the role of social autonomous agents. An agent type can play various social roles and the society diagram can highlight social dimensions of the biological and artificial cells. Immune cells are biological entities using receptors for receiving inputs from the environment. They react on stimuli according to specific rules. Effecting interactions are represented by the perceptor-effector diagram. It represents sensors of autonomous agents and means for sending feedbacks into the environment. Immune cells can be viewed as entities able to offer and use services. The service diagram represents entity types as social entities in the service-based context. The mental diagram is useful only if biological entities are perceived as systems having mental states (believes, goals or plans). Relations between entity types and mental states are represented by mental associations or mental responsibilities. Mental attitude is usually characteristic for people, not for immune cells. On the other hand, immune cells lives in communities and behave proactively or competitively towards goals and plans fulfilment. The mental diagram can highlight this aspect of immune cells. Interactions between immune cells can be represented by the protocol communication diagram. If the immune cells are represented as social entities, the protocol communication diagram can include social roles and model changes in social roles during the life of the immune cell.

Actual attempts in the research in computational immunology combine more approaches together for development of hybrid systems that could improve representation of processes occurring in different scales of organisation of biological system. Research in computational immunology has some difficulties. At least some of them could be overcome with intensive communication and teamwork between theoretical or experimental immunologists and "modellers" for development of valid and useful computational models producing data that are comparable to behaviour of biological system.

11. BIBLIOGRAPHY

ABBAS, A. K. & LICHTMAN, A. H. H. 2010. Basic Immunology: Functions and Disorders of the Immune System, Saunders.

ABBAS, A. K., LICHTMAN, A. H. H. & PILLAI, S. 2011. *Cellular and Molecular Immunology: with STUDENT CONSULT Online Access*, Elsevier Health Sciences.

ALDEN, K. 2012. Simulation and Statistical Techniques to Explore Lymphoid Tissue Organogenesis. Available: http://etheses.whiterose.ac.uk/3220/

ALDEN, K., READ, M., TIMMIS, J., ANDREWS, P. S., VEIGA-FERNANDES, H., COLES, M. 2013. Spartan: A Comprehensive Tool for Understanding Uncertainty in Simulations of Biological Systems. *PLoS Comput Biol 9*, 1-9.

ALDEN, K., TIMMIS, J., READ, M., ANDREWS, P. S., VEIGA-FERNANDES, H., COLES, M. 2012. Pairing experimentation and computational modeling to understand the role of tissue inducer cells in the development of lymphoid organs. *Front Immunol 3*, 172, 1-20.

ALEXANDER, H. K. & WAHL, L. M. 2011. Self-tolerance and autoimmunity in a regulatory T cell model. *Bull Math Biol 73*, 33-71.

ANDREWS, P. S., POLACK, F. A., SAMPSON, A. T., STEPHNEY, S. TIMMIS, J. 2010. The CoSMoS Process. Available: http://www-users.cs.york.ac.uk/susan/bib/ss/nonstd/tr453.htm

ANDREWS, P. S., STEPNEY, S., HOVERD, T., POLACK, F. A. C., SAMPSON, A. T., TIMMIS, J., HOVERD, T. CoSMoS process, models, and metamodels. *Proceedings of the 2011 Workshop on Complex Systems Modelling and Simulation*, France, August 2011, 1-13. Available: http://www-users.cs.york.ac.uk/susan/bib/ss/nonstd/cosmos11-meta.htm

ARLOW, J. & NEUSTADT, I. 2005. UML 2 and the Unified Process: Practical Object-Oriented Analysis and Design, Pearson Education.

ASHBURNER, M., BALL, C. A., BLAKE, J. A., BOTSTEIN D., BUTLER, H. CHERRY, J. M., DAVIS A. P., DOLINSKY, K., DWIGHT, S. S., EPPIG, J. T., HARRIS, M. A., HILL, D. P., ISSEL-TARVER, L., KASARSKIS, A., LEWIS, S. MATESE, J. C., RICHARDSON, J. E., RINGWALD, M., RUBIN, G. M., SHERLOCK, G. 2000. Gene ontology: tool for the unification of biology. The Gene Ontology Consortium. *Nat Genet* 25, 25-29.

AUSUBEL, D. P. 1963. The psychology of meaningful verbal learning, Grune & Stratton.

BAJENOFF, M., EGEN. J. G., KOO, L. Y., LAUGIER, J. P., BRAU, F., CLAICHENHAUS, N., GERMAIN, R. N. 2006. Stromal cell networks regulate lymphocyte entry, migration, and territoriality in lymph nodes. *Immunity* 25, 989-1001.

BANERJEE, S. & MOSES, M. 2009. A Hybrid Agent Based and Differential Equation Model of Body Size Effects on Pathogen Replication and Immune System Response. *In:* ANDREWS, P., TIMMIS, J., OWENS, N. L., AICKELIN, U., HART, E., HONE, A. & TYRRELL, A. (eds.) *Artificial Immune Systems.* Springer Berlin Heidelberg.

BEAUCHEMIN, C. 2002. Modelling the Immune System. Available: http://citeseerx.ist.psu.edu/viewdoc/summary?doi=10.1.1.118.6958

BELKACEM, K. & FOUNDIL, C. 2012. An AnyLogic Agent Based Model for the Lymph Node Lymphocytes First Humoral Immune Response. *International Conference on Bioinformatics and Computational Biology* Singapore: IACSIT Press, 163-169.

BELTMAN, J. B., MARÉE, A. F., LANCH, J. N., MILLER, M. J., DE BOER, R. J. 2007. Lymph node topology dictates T cell migration behavior. *J Exp Med,* 204, 771-780.

BERNASCHI, M. & CASTIGLIONE, F. 2001. Design and implementation of an immune system simulator. *Comput Biol Med,* 31, 303-331.

BERSINI, H. & VARELA, F. 1991. Hints for adaptive problem solving gleaned from immune networks. *In:* SCHWEFEL, H.-P. & MÄNNER, R. (eds.) *Parallel Problem Solving from Nature.* Springer Berlin Heidelberg.

BEZZI, M. & CELLADA, F. 1997. The Transition between Immune and Disease States in a Cellular Automaton Model of Clonal Immune Response. *Physica A,* 145-163.

BORNBERG-BAUER, E. & PATON, N. W. 2002. Conceptual data modelling for bioinformatics. *Briefings in Bioinformatics 3,* 166-180.

BORST, W. N. 1997. *Construction of Engineering Ontologies for Knowledge Sharing and Reuse.* PhD thesis, Universiteit Twente. Available: http://doc.utwente.nl/17864/

CAHALAN, M. D. & PARKER, I. 2005. Close encounters of the first and second kind: T-DC and T-B interactions in the lymph node. *Semin Immunol 17,* 442-451.

CARTER, J. H. 2000. The Immune System as a Model for Pattern Recognition and Classification. *Journal of the American Medical Informatics Association : JAMIA*, 7, 28-41.

CASTIGLIONE, F., DUCA, K., JARRAH, A., LAUBENBACHER, R., HOCHBERG, D., THORLEY-LAWSON, D.. 2007. Simulating Epstein-Barr virus infection with C-ImmSim. *Bioinformatics 23*, 1371-1377.

CASTRO, L. N. D. & TIMMIS, J. 2003. Artificial immune systems as a novel soft computing paradigm. *Soft Computing 7*, 526-544.

CELADA, F. & SEIDEN, P. E. 1992. A computer model of cellular interactions in the immune system. *Immunol Today 13*, 56-62.

CERVENKA, R., GREENWOOD, D., TRENCANSKY, I. 2006. The AML Approach to Modeling Autonomic Systems. Autonomic and Autonomous Systems. ICAS '06. Whitestein Technologies. Silicon Valley, USA, 29-29.

CERVENKA, R. & TRENCANSKY, I. 2007. The Agent Modeling Language - AML: A Comprehensive Approach to Modeling Multi-Agent Systems, Springer-Verlag New York Incorporated.

CHAPLAIN, M. A. J., LACHOWICZ, M., SZYMAŃSKA, Z. & WRZOSEK, D. 2011. Mathematical modelling of cancer invasion: The importance of cell-cell adhesion and cell-matrix adhesion. *Mathematical Models and Methods in Applied Sciences 21*, 719-743.

COAKLEY, S., SMALLWOOD, R., HOLCOMBE, M. 2006. Using X-Machines as a formal basis for describing agents in agent-based modelling. Agent-Directed Simulation, SpringSim 06, 33-40.

COELLO, C. C., RIVERA, D. C., CORTÉS, N. C. 2003. Use of an Artificial Immune System for Job Shop Scheduling. *In:* TIMMIS, J., BENTLEY, P. & HART, E. (eds.) *Artificial Immune Systems.* Springer Berlin Heidelberg.

COHEN, I. R. 2007. Real and artificial immune systems: computing the state of the body. *Nat Rev Immunol 7*, 569-574.

CUELLAR, A., NIELSEN, P., HALSTEAD, M., BULLIVANT, D., NICKERSON, D., HEDLEY, W., NELSON, M., LLOYD, C. 2006. *CellML 1.1 Specification* [Online]. Available: http://www.cellml.org/specifications/cellml_1.1

CUTELLO, V., NICOSIA, G., PAVONE, M., TIMMIS, J. 2007. An Immune Algorithm for Protein Structure Prediction on Lattice Models. *Evolutionary Computation, IEEE Transactions on Evol. Comp. 11*, 101-117.

CYSTER, J. G. & SCHWAB, S. R. 2012. Sphingosine-1-phosphate and lymphocyte egress from lymphoid organs. *Annu Rev Immunol 30*, 69-94.

DASGUPTA, D. & NINO, F. 2008. *Immunological Computation: Theory and Applications*, Auerbach Publications.

DE CASTRO, L. N. 2006. Fundamentals of Natural Computing: Basic Concepts, Algorithms, and Applications, Taylor & Francis.

DE CASTRO, L. N. & TIMMIS, J. 2002. Artificial Immune Systems: A New Computational Intelligence Approach, Springer.

DE CASTRO, L. N. & VON ZUBEN, F. J. 2000. The Clonal Selection Algorithm with Engineering Applications. GECCO'00, Workshop on Artificial Immune Systems and Their Applications, 36-37.

DELVES, P. J. [N. d.]. Lymphatic System: Helping Defend Against Infection In: IMM_LYMPHATIC_SYSTEM (ed.). Available: http://www.merckmanuals.com/home/immune-disorders/biology-of-the-immune-system/overview-of-the-immune-system

DROOP, A., GARNETT, P., POLACK, F. A. C., STEPHNEY, S. 2011. Multiple model simulation: modelling cell division and differentiation in the prostate. *Proceedings of the 2011 Workshop on Complex Systems Modelling and Simulation*. Liniver Press, 79-112.

FARMER, J. D., PACKARD, N. H., PERELSON, A. S. 1986. The immune system, adaptation, and machine learning. *Physica D: Nonlinear Phenomena 22*, 187-204.

FINNEY, A. & HUCKA, M. 2003. Systems biology markup language: Level 2 and beyond. *Biochem Soc Trans 31*, 1472-1473.

FLUGGE, A. J., TIMMIS, J., ANDREWS, P., MOORE, J., KAYE, P. 2009. Modelling and simulation of granuloma formation in visceral leishmaniasis. Congress on Evolutionary Computation, Trondheim, Norway. CEC '09, 18-21 May 2009, 3052-3059.

FOWLER, M. 2003. UML Distilled: A Brief Guide to the Standard Object Modeling Language, Addison-Wesley Longman Publishing Co., Inc.

FRANZOLINI, J. & OLIVIER, D. 2009. Self-Organization in an Artificial Immune Network System. *In:* BERTELLE, C., DUCHAMP, G. E. & KADRI-DAHMANI, H. (eds.) *Complex Systems and Self-organization Modelling*. Springer Berlin Heidelberg.

FUNAHASHI, A., MOROHASHI, M., MATSUOKA, Y., JOURAKU, A., KITANO, H. 2007. CellDesigner: A Graphical Biological Network Editor and Workbench Interfacing Simulator. *In:* CHOI, S. (ed.) *Introduction to Systems Biology*. Humana Press.

GARRETT, S. M. 2005. How Do We Evaluate Artificial Immune Systems? *Evol. Comput. 13*, 145-177.

GARSHOL, L. M. 2006. *The Linear Topic Map Notation* [Online]. Ontopia.net. Available: http://www.ontopia.net/download/ltm.html

GIRARD, J. P., MOUSSION, C. & FORSTER, R. 2012. HEVs, lymphatics and homeostatic immune cell trafficking in lymph nodes. *Nat Rev Immunol 12*, 762-773.

GOODMAN, D., BOGGESS, L. & WATKINS, A. 2002. Artificial immune system classification of multiple-class problems. *Proceedings of the artificial neural networks in engineering ANNIE 2*, 179-183.

GRAY, P. M., PATON, N. W., KEMP, G. J. & FOTHERGILL, J. E. 1990. An object-oriented database for protein structure analysis. *Protein Eng, 3*, 235-243.

GREAVES, R., READ, M., TIMMIS, J., ANDREWS, P. & KUMAR, V. 2012. Extending an Established Simulation: Exploration of the Possible

Effects Using a Case Study in Experimental Autoimmune Encephalomyelitis. *In:* LONES, M., SMITH, S., TEICHMANN, S., NAEF, F., WALKER, J. & TREFZER, M. (eds.) *Information Processign in Cells and Tissues.* Springer Berlin Heidelberg.

GREENSMITH, J., AICKELIN, U. & CAYZER, S. 2005. Introducing Dendritic Cells as a Novel Immune-Inspired Algorithm for Anomaly Detection. *In:* JACOB, C., PILAT, M., BENTLEY, P. & TIMMIS, J. (eds.) *Artificial Immune Systems.* Springer Berlin Heidelberg.

GREENSMITH, J., WHITBROOK, A. & AICKELIN, U. 2010. Artificial immune systems. *Handbook of Metaheuristics.* Springer US.

GRILO, A., CAETANO, A. & ROSA, A. 2002. Immune System Simulation through a Complex Adaptive System Model. *In:* ROY, R., KÖPPEN, M., OVASKA, S., FURUHASHI, T. & HOFFMANN, F. (eds.) *Soft Computing and Industry.* Springer London.

GRUBER, T. R. 1993. A translation approach to portable ontology specifications. *Knowl. Acquis. 5,* 199-220.

GUO, Z. & TAY, J. 2007. A Hybrid Agent-Based Model of Chemotaxis. *In:* SHI, Y., VAN ALBADA, G., DONGARRA, J. & SLOOT, P. A. (eds.) *Computational Science – ICCS 2007.* Springer Berlin Heidelberg.

HARDY, S. & ROBILLARD, P. N. 2004. Modeling and simulation of molecular biology systems using petri nets: modeling goals of various approaches. *J Bioinform Comput Biol 2,* 595-613.

HAREL, D. 1987. Statecharts: A visual formalism for complex systems. *Sci. Comput. Program. 8,* 231-274.

HART, E., DAVOUDANI, D. & MCEWAN, C. 2007. Immunological inspiration for building a new generation of autonomic systems. *Proceedings of the 1st international conference on Autonomic computing and communication systems.* Rome, Italy: ICST (Institute for Computer Sciences, Social-Informatics and Telecommunications Engineering), 1-10.

HEDLEY, W. & NELSON, M. 2001. *CellML 1.0 Specification* [Online]. Available: http://www.cellml.org/specifications/cellml_1.0

HEDLEY, W. J., NELSON, M. R., BELLIVANT, D. P. & NIELSEN, P. F. 2001. A short introduction to CellML. *Philosophical Transactions of the Royal Society of London A: Mathematical, Physical and Engineering Sciences 359,* 1073-1089.

HENRICKSON, S. E. & VON ANDRIAN, U. H. 2007. Single-cell dynamics of T-cell priming. *Curr Opin Immunol 19,* 249-258.

HOFMEYR, S. A. & FORREST, S. 1999. Immunity by Design: An Artificial Immune System. *In:* BANZHAF, W., DAIDA, J., EIBEN, A. E., GARZON, M. H., HONAVAR, V., JAKIELA, M. & SMITH, R. E., eds. Proceedings of the Genetic and Evolutionary Computation Conference, 13-17 July 1999 Orlando, Florida, USA. Morgan Kaufmann, 1289-1296.

HOFMEYR, S. A. & FORREST, S. A. 2000. Architecture for an Artificial Immune System. *Evol. Comput. 8,* 443-473.

HUCKA, M., FINNEY, A., SAURO, H. M., BOLOURI, H., DOYLE, J. C., KITANO, H., FORUM: A. T. R. O. T. S., ARKIN, A. P., BORNSTEIN, B. J., BRAY, D., CORNISH-BOWDEN, A., CUELLAR, A. A., DRONOV, S., GILLES, E. D., GINKEL, M., GOR, V., GORYANIN, I. I., HEDLEY, W. J., HODGMAN, T. C., HOFMEYR, J.-H., HUNTER, P. J., JUTY, N. S., KASBERGER, J. L., KREMLING, A., KUMMER, U., LE NOVÈRE, N., LOEW, L. M., LUCIO, D., MENDES, P., MINCH, E., MJOLSNESS, E. D., NAKAYAMA, Y., NELSON, M. R., NIELSEN, P. F., SAKURADA, T., SCHAFF, J. C., SHAPIRO, B. E., SHIMIZU, T. S., SPENCE, H. D., STELLING, J., TAKAHASHI, K., TOMITA, M., WAGNER, J. & WANG, J. 2003. The systems biology markup language (SBML): a medium for representation and exchange of biochemical network models. *Bioinformatics 19*, 524-531.

HUERTA, M., DOWNING, G. & SETO, B. 2000. NIH Working Definition and Computational Biology. Available: www.bisti.nih.gov/docs/CompuBioDef.pdf

HUNT, J. E. & COOKE, D. E. 1996. Learning using an artificial immune system. *Journal of Network and Computer Applications 19*, 189-212.

HUSÁKOVÁ, M. 2009. Artificial Immune Network Model in NetLogo. *International Conference on Informatics*. Department of Computers and Informatics FEEI TU of Košice, Slovakia, Elfa, 2009, pp. 233 - 238. ISBN 978-80-8086-126-1.

HUSÁKOVÁ, M. 2010. Artificial immune system model based on OWL ontology. *Znalosti 2010*. Jindřichův Hradec: Vysoká škola ekonomická, 211 - 214. ISBN 978-80-245-1636-3.

HUSÁKOVÁ, M. 2014. Dealing with Complexity in Computational Immunology. *In*: BÖHMOVÁ, L. & PAVLÍČEK, A. (eds.) *System approaches 2014*. Prague: University of Economics, Publishing Oeconomica, 74-78.

HUSÁKOVÁ, M. 2015a. Combating Infectious Diseases with Computational Immunology. *In*: NUNEZ M., N. N., -T., CAMACHO D., TRAWINSKI, B. (ed.) *Computational Collective Intelligence Technologies and Applications*. Madrid: Springer-Verlag (*in press*).

HUSÁKOVÁ, M. 2015b. The Usage of the Agent Modeling Language for Modeling Complexity of the Immune System. *In*: BARBUCHA, D., NGUYEN, N. T. & BATUBARA, J. (eds.) *New Trends in Intelligent Information and Database Systems*. Springer International Publishing, 323-332.

HUSÁKOVÁ, M. 2015c. Using Concept Maps in Education of Immunological Computation and Computational Immunology. *In*: NUNEZ M., N. N.-T., CAMACHO D., TRAWINSKI, B. (ed.) *Computational Collective Intelligence Technologies and Applications*. Madrid: Springer-Verlag, (*in press*)

ICHIKAWA, S., KUBOSHIKI, S., ISHIGURO, A. & UCHIKAWA, Y. 1998. A method of gait coordination of hexapod robots using immune networks. *Artificial Life and Robotics 2*, 19-23.

ISO 2008. ISO 13250-2: Topic Maps — Data Model. ISO. Available: http://www.isotopicmaps.org/sam/

JACOB, C., LITORCO, J. & LEE, L. 2004. Immunity Through Swarms: Agent-Based Simulations of the Human Immune System. *In:* NICOSIA, G., CUTELLO, V., BENTLEY, P. & TIMMIS, J. (eds.) *Artificial Immune Systems.* Springer Berlin Heidelberg, 400-412.

JERNE, N. K. 1974a. Clonal selection in a lymphocyte network. *Soc Gen Physiol Ser 29*, 39-48.

JERNE, N. K. 1974b. Towards a network theory of the immune system. *Ann Immunol (Paris)*, 125C, 373-389.

KATAKAI, T., HARA, T., LEE, J.-H., GONDA, H., SUGAI, M. & SHIMIZU, A. 2004. A novel reticular stromal structure in lymph node cortex: an immuno-platform for interactions among dendritic cells, T cells and B cells. *International Immunology 16*, 1133-1142.

KERNBACH, S., MEISTER, E., SCHLACHTER, F., JEBENS, K., SZYMANSKI, M., LIEDKE, J., LANERI, D., WINKLER, L., SCHMICKL, T., THENIUS, R., CORRADI, P. & RICOTTI, L. 2008. Symbiotic robot organisms: REPLICATOR and SYMBRION projects. *Proceedings of the 8th Workshop on Performance Metrics for Intelligent Systems.* Gaithersburg, Maryland: ACM, 62-69.

KHAN, S., MAKKENA, R., MCGEARY, F., DECKER, K., GILLIS, W. & SCHMIDT, C. 2003. A multi-agent system for the quantitative simulation of biological networks. *Proceedings of the second international joint conference on Autonomous agents and multiagent systems.* Melbourne, Australia: ACM, 385-392.

KIM, P. S. & LEE, P. P. 2012. Modeling protective anti-tumor immunity via preventative cancer vaccines using a hybrid agent-based and delay differential equation approach. *PLoS Comput Biol 8*. Available: http://www.ploscompbiol.org/article/metrics/info%3Adoi%2F10.1371%2Fjournal.pcbi.1002742;jsessionid=D6BBC0E1892D5E2D2FB1C6C93B7A67C9

KITANO, H. 2003. A Graphical Notation for Biological Networks. *BioSilico 1*, 169-176. Available: http://citeseerx.ist.psu.edu/viewdoc/summary?doi=10.1.1.541.4169

KITANO, H., MATSUOKA, Y., FUNAHASHI, A. & ODA, K. [N. d.]. *The Process Diagram: Rationale and Definition* [Online]. The Systems Biology Institute. Available: http://www.celldesigner.org/documents/ProcessDiagram.html

KOESTLER, A. 1967. *The ghost in the machine*, Macmillan.

KOHN, K. W. 1999. Molecular interaction map of the mammalian cell cycle control and DNA repair systems. *Mol Biol Cell 10*, 2703-2734.

KONIG, M., DRAGER, A. & HOLZHUTTER, H. G. 2012. CySBML: a Cytoscape plugin for SBML. *Bioinformatics 28*, 2402-2403.
KRAUSE, F., SCHULZ, M., RIPKENS, B., FLÖTTMANN, M., KRANTZ, M., KLIPP, E. & HANDORF, T. 2013. Biographer: web-based editing and rendering of SBGN compliant biochemical networks. *Bioinformatics 29*, 1467-1468.
KRAUSE, F., UHLENDORF, J., LUBITZ, T., SCHULZ, M., KLIPP, E. & LIEBERMEISTER, W. 2010. Annotation and merging of SBML models with semanticSBML. *Bioinformatics 26*, 421-422.
KUGLER, H., LARJO, A. & HAREL, D. 2010. Biocharts: a visual formalism for complex biological systems. *Journal of The Royal Society Interface 7*, 1015-1024.
LACY, L. W. 2005. Owl: Representing Information Using the Web Ontology Language, Trafford.
LACY, L. W., YOUNGBLOOD, S. & MIGHT, R. 2001. Developing a Consensus Perspective on Conceptual Models for Simulation Systems. *Spring Simulation Interoperability Workshop.*
LARMAN, C. 2004. Applying UML and Patterns: An Introduction to Object-Oriented Analysis and Design and Iterative Development, Prentice Hall.
LAVELLE, C., P., B., BERRY, H. & BESLON, G. 2012. *Roadmap Complex Systems: from molecule to organism* [Online]. Available: http://immunocomplexit.net/
LE NOVERE, N., HUCKA, M., MI, H., MOODIE, S., SCHREIBER, F., SOROKIN, A., DEMIR, E., WEGNER, K., ALADJEM, M. I., WIMALARATNE, S. M., BERGMAN, F. T., GAUGES, R., GHAZAL, P., KAWAJI, H., LI, L., MATSUOKA, Y., VILLEGER, A., BOYD, S. E., CALZONE, L., COURTOT, M., DOGRUSOZ, U., FREEMAN, T. C., FUNAHASHI, A., GHOSH, S., JOURAKU, A., KIM, S., KOLPAKOV, F., LUNA, A., SAHLE, S., SCHMIDT, E., WATTERSON, S., WU, G., GORYANIN, I., KELL, D. B., SANDER, C., SAURO, H., SNOEP, J. L., KOHN, K. & KITANO, H. 2009. The Systems Biology Graphical Notation. *Nat Biotechnol 27*, 735-741.
LE NOVÈRE, N., MOODIE, S., SOROKIN, A., HUCKA, M., MI, H., SCHREIBER, F., DEMIR, E., MATSUOKA, Y., WEJNER, K. & KITANO, H. 2008. Systems Biology Graphical Notation: Process Description language Level 1, Version 1.0. COMBINE web. Available: http://co.mbine.org/specifications/sbgn.pd.level-1
LE NOVÈRE, N., MOODIE, S., SOROKIN, A., SCHREIBER, F. & MI, H. 2009. Systems Biology Graphical Notation: Entity Relationship language Level 1, Version 1.0. COMBINE web. Available: http://co.mbine.org/specifications/sbgn.er.level-1.version-1.2
LEANDRO NUNES DE, C. & FERNANDO, J. V. Z. 2002. aiNet: An Artificial Immune Network for Data Analysis. *In:* HUSSEIN, A. A., CHARLES, S. N. & RUHUL, S. (eds.) *Data Mining: A Heuristic Approach.* Hershey, PA, USA: IGI Global.

LI, L. & RONG, Q.-M. 2009. Implementation of Clustering Algorithm Using Artificial Immune System. Database Technology and Applications 2009, 25-26 April, 2009. 275-278.

LIKIC, V. A., MCCONVILLE, M. J., LITHGOW, T. & BACIC, A. 2010. Systems biology: the next frontier for bioinformatics. *Adv Bioinformatics.* No. 268925. Hindawi Publishing Corp.

LIU, B., ZHANG, J., TAN, P. Y., HSU, D., BLOM, A. M., LEONG, B., SETHI, S., HO, B., DING, J. L. & THIAGARAJAN, P. S. 2011. A Computational and Experimental Study of the Regulatory Mechanisms of the Complement System. *PLoS Comput Biol 7.* Available: http://journals.plos.org/ploscompbiol/article?id=10.1371/journal.pcbi.1001059

LLOYD, C. M., HALSTEAD, M. D. & NIELSEN, P. F. 2004. CellML: its future, present and past. *Prog Biophys Mol Biol 85,* 433-450.

LUND, O., NIELSEN, M., LUNDEGAARD, C., KESMIR, C., S, & BRUNAK, R. 2005. *Immunological Bioinformatics (Computational Molecular Biology),* The MIT Press.

MALIM, M. R., KHADER, A. T. & MUSTAFA, A. 2006. Artificial immune algorithms for university timetabling. *Proceedings of the 6th international conference on practice and theory of automated timetabling,* 234-245.

MASOUDI-NEJAD, A. & MESHKIN, A. 2014. Cancer modeling: The holonic agent-based approach. *Semin Cancer Biol.* DOI: 10.1016/j.semcancer.2014.02.008.

MCCARTHY, J. 1987. Circumscription—a form of non-monotonic reasoning. *In:* MATTHEW, L. G. (ed.) *Readings in nonmonotonic reasoning.* Morgan Kaufmann Publishers Inc.

MCGILLEN, J. B., MARTIN, N. K., ROBEY, I. F., GAFFNEY, E. A. & MAINI, P. K. 2012. Application of mathematical analysis to tumour acidity modelling. Available: https://people.maths.ox.ac.uk/maini/PKM%20publications/349.pdf

MEIER-SCHELLERSHEIM, M. & MACK, G. 1999. Simulator SIMMUNE, a tool for stimulating and analyzing immune system behaviour. Available: http://citeseerx.ist.psu.edu/viewdoc/summary;jsessionid=5E5342A2FE8E44A77DE86C7E0F9CA99C?doi=10.1.1.342.7503

MELLOR, S. J. 2004. *Agile MDA* [Online]. Available: http://www.omg.org/mda/mda_files/AgileMDA.pdf

MI, H., SCHREIBER, F., LE NOVÈRE, N., MOODIE, S. & SOROKIN, A. 2009. Systems Biology Graphical Notation: Activity Flow language Level 1, Version 1.0. COMBINE web. Available: http://co.mbine.org/specifications/sbgn.af.level-1

MILES, R. & HAMILTON, K. 2006. *Learning UML 2.0,* O'Reilly Media, Inc.

MILLER, M. J., HEJAZI, A. S., WEI, S. H., CAHALAN, M. D. & PARKER, I. 2004. T cell repertoire scanning is promoted by dynamic dendritic cell behavior and random T cell motility in the lymph node. *Proc Natl Acad Sci USA 101,* 998-1003.

MILLER, M. J., WEI, S. H., PARKER, I. & CAHALAN, M. D. 2002. Two-photon imaging of lymphocyte motility and antigen response in intact lymph node. *Science* 296, 1869-1873.

MOODIE, S. L., SOROKIN, A., GROYANIN, I. & GHAZAL, P. 2006. A Graphica Notation to describe the Logical Interactions of Biological Pathways. *Journal of Integrative Bioinformatics 3*, p. 11.

MOORE, J. W., MOYO, D., BEATTIE, L., ANDREWS, P. S., TIMMIS, J. & KAYE, P. M. 2013. Functional complexity of the Leishmania granuloma and the potential of in silico modeling. *Front Immunol, 4*, 35. Available: http://journal.frontiersin.org/article/10.3389/fimmu.2013.00035/full

MORARU, I. I., SCHAFF, J. C., SLEPCHENKO, B. M., BLINOV, M., MORGAN, F., LAKSHMINARAYANA, A., GAO, F., LI, Y. & LOEW, L. M. 2008. The Virtual Cell Modeling and Simulation Software Environment. *IET systems biology 2*, 352-362.

MOROWITZ, H. J. & SINGER, J. L. 1995. *The Mind, the Brain, and Complex Adaptive Systems*, Addison-Wesley Publishing Company.

MÜLLER, H. A. 2006. Autonomic Computing: Software Architecture Technology. Carnegie Mellon University.

MURPHY, K. P., TRAVERS, P., WALPORT, M. & JANEWAY, C. 2008. *Janeway's Immunobiology*, Garland Science.

NAIR, A. S. 2007. Computational Biology and Bioinformatics: A Gentle Overview. *Communications of the Computer Society of India, 12*.

NANCE, R. 1994. The Conical Methodology and the evolution of simulation model development. *Annals of Operations Research 53*, 1-45.

NOVAK, J. 1990. Concept maps and Vee diagrams: two metacognitive tools to facilitate meaningful learning. *Instructional Science 19*, 29-52.

NOVAK, J. D. 2002. Meaningful learning: The essential factor for conceptual change in limited or inappropriate propositional hierarchies leading to empowerment of learners. *Science Education 86*, 548-571.

NOVAK, J. D. & CAÑAS, A. J. 2006. The Theory Underlying Concept Maps and How to Construct Them. Available: http://web.stanford.edu/dept/SUSE/projects/ireport/articles/concept_maps/The%20Theory%20Underlying%20Concept%20Maps.pdf

OKADA, T. & CYSTER, J. G. 2007. CC chemokine receptor 7 contributes to Gi-dependent T cell motility in the lymph node. *J Immunol 178*, 2973-2978.

ONTOPIA Ontopia. [N. d.] ontopia.net: Ontopia. Available: http://www.ontopia.net/

PAINTER, K. J. 2009. Continuous models for cell migration in tissues and applications to cell sorting via differential chemotaxis. *Bull Math Biol 71*, 1117-1147.

PATON, N. W., KHAN, S. A., HAYES, A., MOUSSOUNI, F., BRASS, A., EILBECK, K., GOBLE, C. A., HUBBARD, S. J. & OLIVER, S. G. 2000. Conceptual modelling of genomic information. *Bioinformatics 16*, 548-557.

PERELSON, A. S. & OSTER, G. F. 1979. Theoretical studies of clonal selection: minimal antibody repertoire size and reliability of self-non-self discrimination. *J Theor Biol 81*, 645-670.

PÉREZ, P. P. G., GERSHENSON, C., CÁRDENAS-GARCÍA, M. & LAGUNEZ-OTERO, J. 2002. Modelling intracellular signalling networks using behaviour-based systems and the blackboard architecture. CoRR, cs.MA/0211029. Available: http://arxiv.org/abs/cs.MA/0211029

PILONE, D. & PITMAN, N. 2005. *UML 2.0 in a Nutshell*, O'Reilly Media.

PINNEY, J. W., WESTHEAD, D. R. & MCCONKEY, G. A. 2003. Petri Net representations in systems biology. *Biochem Soc Trans 31*, 1513-1515.

POGSON, M., HOLCOMBE, M., SMALLWOOD, R. & QWARNSTROM, E. 2008. Introducing Spatial Information into Predictive NF-κB Modelling – An Agent-Based Approach. *PLoS ONE 3*, e2367. Available: http://journals.plos.org/plosone/article?id=10.1371/journal.pone.0002367

RAFFAT, S. K. 2012. Human Biological Viruses Ontology. *Research Journal of Recent Sciences 1*, 10, 45-50.

RAPIN, N., LUND, O., BERNASCHI, M. & CASTIGLIONE, F. 2010. Computational Immunology Meets Bioinformatics: The Use of Prediction Tools for Molecular Binding in the Simulation of the Immune System. *PLoS ONE 5*, e9862. Available: http://journals.plos.org/plosone/article?id=10.1371/journal.pone.0009862

READ, M., ANDREWS, P., TIMMIS, J. & KUMAR, V. 2009. A Domain Model of Experimental Autoimmune Encephalomyelitis. 2nd Workshop on Complex Systems Modelling and Simulation 2009. 9-44.

REDDY, V. N., MAVROVOUNIOTIS, M. L. & LIEBMAN, M. N. 1993. Petri net representations in metabolic pathways. *Proc Int Conf Intell Syst Mol Biol 1*, 328-336.

REN, L. H., DING, Y. S., SHEN, Y. Z. & ZHANG, X. F. 2008. Multi-agent-based bio-network for systems biology: protein-protein interaction network as an example. *Amino Acids 35*, 565-572.

ROBINSON, P. N. & BAUER, S. 2011. *Introduction to Bio-Ontologies*, Taylor & Francis.

ROUSSEY, C., PINET, F., KANG, M. & CORCHO, O. 2011. An Introduction to Ontologies and Ontology Engineering. *Ontologies in Urban Development Projects*. Springer London.

SACKMANN, A., HEINER, M. & KOCH, I. 2006. Application of Petri net based analysis techniques to signal transduction pathways. *BMC Bioinformatics*. Available: http://www.biomedcentral.com/1471-2105/7/482

SANTOS, E. E., GUO, D., SANTOS, E. & ONESTY, W. 2004. A Multi-Agent System Environment for Modelling Cell and Tissue. *International Conference on Parallel and Distributed Processing Techniques and Applications*. Nevada, Las Vegas: CSREA Press.

SBGNDICTIONARY. [N. d.] *SBGN bricks dictionary* [Online].
sourceforge.net. Available:
http://sbgnbricks.sourceforge.net/sbgnbricks_dictionary.html
SECKER, A., FREITAS, A. A. & TIMMIS, J. 2003. AISEC: an artificial
immune system for e-mail classification. Evolutionary Computation,
CEC '03, 8-12 Dec. 2003. 131-138.
SHANNON, P., MARKIEL, A., OZIER, O., BALIGA, N. S., WANG, J. T.,
RAMAGE, D., AMIN, N., SCHWIKOWSKI, B. & IDEKER, T. 2003.
Cytoscape: A Software Environment for Integrated Models of
Biomolecular Interaction Networks. *Genome Research 13*, 2498-2504.
SCHOEBERL, B., EICHLER-JONSSON, C., GILLES, E. D. & MULLER, G.
2002. Computational modeling of the dynamics of the MAP kinase
cascade activated by surface and internalized EGF receptors. *Nat
Biotechnol 20*, 370-375.
SMALLWOOD, R. & HOLCOMBE, M. 2006. The Epitheliome Project:
multiscale agent-based modeling of epithelial cells. Proceedings of the
2006 IEEE International Symposium on Biomedical Imaging: From
Nano to Macro, 6-9 April 2006, 816-819.
SMOLEN, P. D., BAXTER, D. A. & BYRNE, J. H. 2003. Modeling and
Analysis of Intracellular Signaling Pathways. *From Molecules to Networks:
An Introduction to Cellular and Molecular Neuroscience*. Academic Press.
SOMPAYRAC, L. 2012. How the Immune System Works, Includes Desktop
Edition, Wiley.
StarUML 2.2 ed. [N. d.]. [Online]. Available: http://staruml.io/
STEPNEY, S., SMITH, R., TIMMIS, J. & TYRRELL, A. 2004. Towards a
Conceptual Framework for Artificial Immune Systems. *In*: NICOSIA, G.,
CUTELLO, V., BENTLEY, P. & TIMMIS, J. (eds.) *Artificial Immune
Systems*. Springer Berlin Heidelberg, 53-64. Available:
http://citeseerx.ist.psu.edu/viewdoc/summary?doi=10.1.1.95.4380
STITES, D. P., TERR, A. I. & PARSLOW, T. G. 1994. *Basic & Clinical
Immunology*, McGraw-Hill Education.
SWERDLIN, N., COHEN, I. R. & HAREL, D. 2008. The Lymph Node B Cell
Immune Response: Dynamic Analysis In-Silico. *Proceedings of the IEEE*,
96, 1421-1443.
TAKAYANAGI, T., KAWAMURA, H. & OHUCHI, A. 2006. Cellular
Automaton Model of a Tumor Tissue Consisting of Tumor Cells,
Cytotoxic T Lymphocytes (CTLs), and Cytokine Produced by CTLs. *IPSJ
Transactions on Mathematical Modeling and Applications 47*, 61-67.
TAO, L., YIWEN, L., HUAN, Y. & JIA, C. An Integrated Artificial Immune
Systems Model Based On Ontology. Intelligent Computation
Technology and Automation (ICICTA), 2008 International Conference
on, 20-22 Oct. 2008. 819-822.
TARAKANOV, A., GONCHAROVA, L. & TARAKANOV, O. 2005. A
Cytokine Formal Immune Network. *In*: CAPCARRÈRE, M., FREITAS,

A., BENTLEY, P., JOHNSON, C. & TIMMIS, J. (eds.) *Advances in Artificial Life*. Springer Berlin Heidelberg.

TIMMIS, J. 2006. Challenges for Artificial Immune Systems. *In:* APOLLONI, B., MARINARO, M., NICOSIA, G. & TAGLIAFERRI, R. (eds.) *Neural Nets*. Springer Berlin Heidelberg, 355-367.

TIMMIS, J. 2007. Artificial immune systems-today and tomorrow. *Journal Natural Computing 6*, 1-18.

TIMMIS, J., ANDREWS, P., OWENS, N. & CLARK, E. 2008. Immune Systems and Computation: An Interdisciplinary Adventure. *In:* CALUDE, C., COSTA, J., FREUND, R., OSWALD, M. & ROZENBERG, G. (eds.) *Unconventional Computing*. Springer Berlin Heidelberg, 8-18.

TIMMIS, J. & NEAL, M. 2001. A resource limited artificial immune system for data analysis. *Knowledge-Based Systems 14*, 121-130.

TIMMIS, J., NEAL, M. & HUNT, J. 2000. An artificial immune system for data analysis. *Biosystems 55*, 143-150.

TODAR, K. [N. d.]. Origin and differentiation of cells of the immune system. *In:* CELLSINDEFENSES75 (ed.). Available: http://textbookofbacteriology.net/adaptive_2.html

TOPA, P. 2006. Towards a Two-Scale Cellular Automata Model of Tumour-Induced Angiogenesis. *In:* EL YACOUBI, S., CHOPARD, B. & BANDINI, S. (eds.) *Cellular Automata*. Springer Berlin Heidelberg, 337-346.

TWYCROSS, J. & AICKELIN, U. 2007. Biological Inspiration for Artificial Immune Systems. *In:* DE CASTRO, L., VON ZUBEN, F. & KNIDEL, H. (eds.) *Artificial Immune Systems*. Springer Berlin Heidelberg, 300-311.

UML Tutorial [n. d.][Online]. SparxSystems homepage. Available: http://www.sparxsystems.com/uml-tutorial.html

USCHOLD, M. & GRUNINGER, M. 1996. Ontologies: principles, methods and applications. *The Knowledge Engineering Review 11*, 43, 93-136. Available: http://citeseerx.ist.psu.edu/viewdoc/summary?doi=10.1.1.111.5903

VON ANDRIAN, U. H. & MEMPEL, T. R. 2003. Homing and cellular traffic in lymph nodes. *Nat Rev Immunol 3*, 867-878.

WALKER, D. C., SOUTHGATE, J., HILL, G., HOLCOMBE, M., HOSE, D. R., WOOD, S. M., MAC NEIL, S. & SMALLWOOD, R. H. 2004. The epitheliome: agent-based modelling of the social behaviour of cells. *Biosystems 76*, 89-100.

WEBB, K. & WHITE, T. 2005. UML as a cell and biochemistry modeling language. *Biosystems 80*, 283-302.

WEI, S. H., PARKER, I., MILLER, M. J. & CAHALAN, M. D. 2003. A stochastic view of lymphocyte motility and trafficking within the lymph node. *Immunol Rev 195*, 136-159.

WHETZEL, P. L., NOY, N. F., SHAH, N. H., ALEXANDER, P. R., NYULAS, C., TUDORACHE, T. & MUSEN, M. A. 2011. BioPortal: enhanced functionality via new Web services from the National Center for

Biomedical Ontology to access and use ontologies in software applications. *Nucleic Acids Research 39*, 541-545. Available: http://www.ncbi.nlm.nih.gov/pmc/articles/PMC3125807/

WILLIAMS, R. A., READ, M., TIMMIS, J., ANDREWS, P. S. & KUMAR, V. 2013. In silico investigation into dendritic cell regulation of CD8Treg mediated killing of Th1 cells in murine experimental autoimmune encephalomyelitis. *BMC Bioinformatics 14*, 9. Available: http://link.springer.com/article/10.1186%2F1471-2105-14-S6-S9

WORBS, T., MEMPEL, T. R., BOLTER, J., VON ANDRIAN, U. H. & FORSTER, R. 2007. CCR7 ligands stimulate the intranodal motility of T lymphocytes in vivo. *J Exp Med 204*, 489-495.

YAMADA, S., SHIONO, S., JOO, A. & YOSHIMURA, A. 2003. Control mechanism of JAK/STAT signal transduction pathway. *FEBS Lett 534*, 190-196.

ZORZENON DOS SANTOS, R. M. & COUTINHO, S. 2001. Dynamics of HIV Infection: A Cellular Automata Approach. *Physical Review Letters 87*, 168102.

12. Subject Index

A

13. Name Index

A

H

J

K

M

N

O

P

R

S

V

14. LIST O FIGURES

15. List of Acronyms

Ab (AB): Antibody
ACL: Agent Communication Language
AF: Activity Flow Language
AIS: Artificial Immune System
AIS-OWL: Artificial Immune System-Ontology Web Language
AML: Agent Modelling Language
APC: Antigen-Presenting Cell
ARTIMMUS: Artificial Murine Multiple Sclerosis Simulation
BCR: B-Cell Receptor
CA: Cellular Automata
CellAK: Cell Assembly Kit
CI: Computational Immunology
CM: Concept map
CoSMoS: Complex Systems Modelling and Simulation
DC: Dendritic Cell
DECAF: Distributed Environment Centered Agent Framework
DNA: Deoxyribonucleic Acid
EAE: Experimental Autoimmune Encephalomyelitis
EBD: Expected Behaviour Diagram
EPN: Edinburgh Pathway Notation
ER: Entity Relationship Language
ERD: Entity-Relationship Diagram
EVL: Experimental Visceral Laishmaniasis
FDC: Follicular Dendritic Cell
FRC: Fibroblastic Reticular Cell
GO: Gene Ontology

HBVO: Human Biological Viruses Ontology
HER: Human Epidermal Growth Factor Receptor
HEV: High Endothelial Venules
HLA: Human Leukocyte Antigen
IC: Immunological Computation
IL: Interleukin
ISO: International Standard Organisation
LTM: Linear Topic Map Notation
MAS: Multi-Agent System
MHC: Major Histocompatibility Complex
MIM: Molecular Interaction Maps
NCBO: National Center for Biomedical Ontology
NIH: National Institutes of Health
NIS: Natural Immune System
NK: Natural Killer
NS: Negative Selection
OBO: Open Biomedical Ontologies, Open Biological and Biomedical Ontologies
ODE: Ordinary Differential Equations
OMG: Object Modelling Group
OMT: Object Modelling Technique
OWL: Ontology Web Language
PD: Process Description Language
PDB: Protein Data Bank
PDE: Partial Differential Equation
PPSIM: Peyer's Patches Simulator
PS: Positive Selection
RDF: Resource Description Framework
RDF(S): Resource Description Framework Schema
S1P: Spingosine-1-Phosphate
SBGN: Systems Biology Graphical Notation
SBML: Systems Biology Markup Language
T_c-cell: $T_{cytotoxic}$-cell
TCR: T-Cell Receptor
T_h-cell: T_{helper}-cell
T_{reg}-cell: $T_{regulatory}$-cell
T_{sup}-cell: $T_{suppressor}$-cell
UML: Unified Modelling Language
VUE: Visual Understanding Environment
XML: Extensible Markup Language

16. APPENDIXES

APPENDIX A: Elements of the Process diagram adopted by CellDesigner 2.0 (Kitano et al. [n. d.])

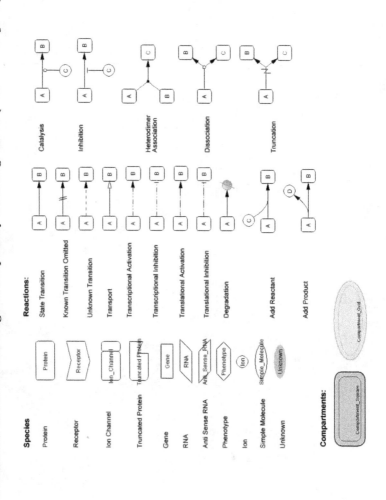

APPENDIX B: Elements of the Process Description Language (Le Novère et al., 2008)

172

APPENDIX C: Elements of the Entity Relationship Language (Le Novère et al., 2009)

SYSTEMS BIOLOGY GRAPHICAL NOTATION ENTITY RELATIONSHIP REFERENCE CARD

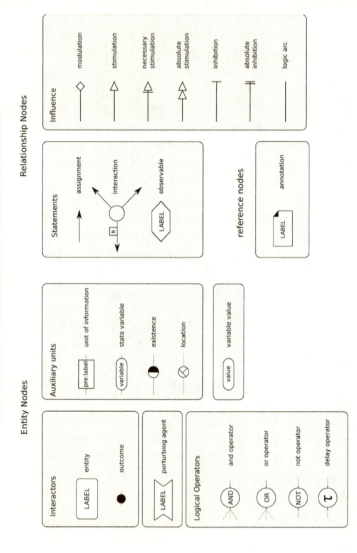

APPENDIX D: Elements of the Activity Flow Language (Mi et al., 2009)

SYSTEMS BIOLOGY GRAPHICAL NOTATION ACTIVITY FLOW DIAGRAM REFERENCE CARD

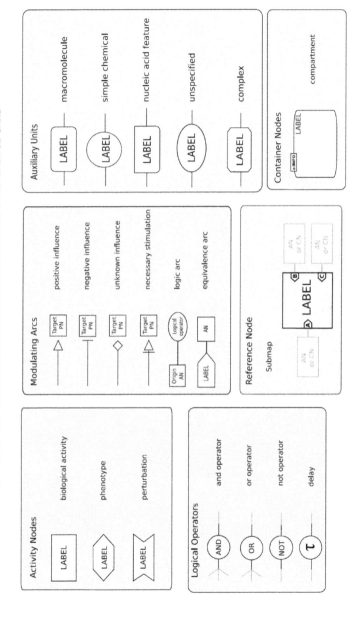